THE BES...
Hilton Head M...
WAS ALRE...
NOW IT'S EVEN ...

The original *Hilton Head Metabolism Diet* showed you
how to increase your body's fat-burning ability and let
you eat lots of delicious good food. Created by a leading
weight-control expert, it made weight loss easy and safe
with no fad foods, unhealthy food restrictions, or unap-
petizing meals. But now, new scientific discoveries make
THE NEW HILTON HEAD METABOLISM DIET
even better—reducing body fat and improving your
overall health. Here's what's new:

- **The exclusive Stair Stepping plan**—based on
  state-of-the-art research, Stair Stepping allows you to
  lose in stages to achieve gradual, permanent weight
  loss and a metabolism that won't slow down.
- **The 10% solution**—the way to use weight loss to
  dramatically improve your overall health and energy
  level
- **Easy-to-learn exercises**—great toning and lean muscle building exercises so you can look trim . . . without being skinny
- **Fast 14-day weight loss meal plan**—Yes! You do
  eat *five* times a day, never feel hungry, and watch fat
  melt away!
- **Genetic research**—find out if you are at risk to suffer obesity as a chronic disease—and what you can do
  about it, right now!

 . . . plus new motivation techniques, exciting recipes,
 weight-training exercise plans, and more!

THE NEW
HILTON HEAD
METABOLISM
DIET

DR. PETER M. MILLER

WARNER BOOKS

A Time Warner Company

WARNER BOOKS EDITION

Cover design by Rachel McClain
Book design by H. Roberts

Warner Books, Inc.
1271 Avenue of the Americas
New York, NY 10020

Visit our Web site at
www.warnerbooks.com

W A Time Warner Company

Printed in the United States of America

First Printing: June, 1996

10 9 8 7 6

For Miller—
With love from Pop-Pete

◼ ◼ ◼

ACKNOWLEDGMENTS

I am greatly indebted to my staff at the Hilton Head Health Institute for their continuing contributions to the content of the New Hilton Head Metabolism Diet. I would especially like to acknowledge the assistance of my wife, Gay, as well as Robert Wright, Fran Gerthoffer, Erich Striegel, and Dr. Roger Sargent in the preparation of this book.

I am particularly grateful to the thousands of men and women who have participated in our programs at the Hilton Head Health Institute and who continue to share their success stories with us.

ACKNOWLEDGMENT

I am greatly indebted to my and in this, for their health insights for their continuing encouragement to the critics of my New Edition and Metabolism Diet. I would especially like to acknowledge the resource of my wife, Gay, as well as Allen, Wendell, Ron Christianson, Jack Siegel, and Dr. James Sargent in the development of this work.

I am particularly grateful to the thousands of men and women who have established fitness programs at the Institute for Aerobic Research and who continue to share their experiences with us.

◼ ◼ ◼
CONTENTS

Chapter 1
◼ ◼ ◼
It's Not Your Fault

If you've tried every new diet developed over the past few years, only to gain your weight back again, you are definitely not alone. Perhaps, more recently, you joined the antidieting movement and found your weight problem getting worse with each passing day. Or you may have adopted a healthier lifestyle by lowering the amount of fat you eat, only to find that you still have trouble losing weight and keeping it off.

If any of these problems describe your battle of the bulge, you are more typical than you realize. You likely feel frustrated and depressed about your weight and simply don't know where to turn.

Your failures are not your fault. You've just been going about it the wrong way. I want you now to forget everything you've ever learned about dieting. I'm going to give you a system of weight control that gives you a fighting chance. One that has helped over *a million* men and women throughout the world. That's how many people purchased my previous book, *The Hilton Head Metabolism Diet.*

This version, *The New Hilton Head Metabolism Diet,* is an improved diet based on the most recent research available. This is not simply another diet but a totally new frame of reference. It is based on the premise that your weight problem is not due simply to a lack of willpower.

Overweight is a complex biological, metabolic, and nutritional disease that requires a specially designed, comprehensive treatment plan. That's right. You must begin to think of your weight problem as a chronic disease. All the latest research points to this conclusion, and it is important for you to remember it.

Your problem is not just a matter of eating too much but of not burning enough calories. While exercise is an important part of the solution, *you actually burn 70 percent of all your calories each day through metabolism and only 30 percent through physical activity.* That's why having a sluggish metabolism makes weight control so difficult. Unless you attack your basic problem of metabolic suppression no diet will ever help you.

How the New Hilton Head Metabolism Diet Was Created

Twenty years ago I founded what has become one of the top health resorts in the world. Unlike a spa, my Hilton Head Health Institute is noted for its professional, scientifically based treatment programs and has served as the proving grounds for the Hilton Head Metabolism Diet.

Even before I started the institute, I had become frustrated by the failure of many of my patients to lose weight. Some would stick strictly to a diet but still prove unable to lose much weight. Others would lose but regain the lost weight within two or three months. It amazed me how people on exactly the same diet and exercise program could differ so much in the results they achieved.

To find a new approach I began listening more closely to my patients' complaints:

"My friend Sally eats anything she wants and never gains an ounce. I can gain six pounds in a holiday weekend."

"But, Doctor, even when I do lose weight, it's a constant struggle to keep from gaining it back. Slim people don't seem to have the same problem."

"I just can't lose weight as easily as other people. Maybe it's my thyroid."

Like many of my colleagues, I assured these people that their problem was not glandular. They simply ate too much. I might even have suspected a complaining patient of trying to use metabolism as an excuse for cheating on the diet.

Fortunately, I began to pay more attention to these complaints. I took them more seriously and began to investigate the differences in individuals' ability to control their weight. I started by examining the records of my patients over the previous years, comparing their eating, exercise, and weight patterns with those of slim people. Next I compiled the results of every major research study comparing weight regulation, eating, exercise, and metabolism in overweight and nonoverweight individuals.

As a result of these investigations, I departed radically from traditional ideas about dieting. I'm now very pleased that I did, because my program has helped so many people over the years.

The evidence in favor of the Hilton Head Metabolism Diet is impressive. The research studies have been there all along. In fact, over the past ten years since the diet was originally developed, more and more experts have come to agree that metabolism is the major key to unlocking the weight control puzzle. I'm pleased to see the evidence mounting to support my ideas, which several years ago were considered controversial.

Study after study verifies the fact that you are overweight because of your failure to burn calories efficiently through metabolism. In most cases, your metabolism is not abnormal, just sluggish. The New Hilton Head Metabolism Diet is designed not merely to help you lose weight but to enable you to change your body chemistry so that weight control becomes easier. In a moment I will explain why you don't burn as many calories as a slim person does and what you can do about it.

YOU WERE RIGHT ALL ALONG

So stop feeling guilty and frustrated. Your difficulty in regulating your weight is not due to laziness or gluttony. You were right all along: You *do* gain weight more easily than slim people. You've been telling people this for years, but they haven't been listening to you. Well, I believe you, and I have evidence to prove the "experts" wrong and you right. Your burden of carrying all that extra weight and taking the blame is over.

I don't want you ever to feel guilty again or let anyone else make you feel guilty about your weight. Doctors, spouses, and friends simply don't understand, especially if they are slim. You don't have to accept the blame anymore. I'm going to liberate you from all this frustration.

A TOTALLY NEW APPROACH

Once you begin my plan you'll realize how different an approach it is to controlling your weight. It's like discovering a medicine that has just been developed to help you manage your chronic disease.

Like those who have already benefited from the Hilton Head Metabolism Diet, you will soon experience the fact that my new system:

- Stimulates your ability to burn fat by naturally increasing your metabolic rate
- Tunes your metabolic engine so that you burn more calories without added effort
- Encourages you to eat *more* meals rather than less
- Gives you three easy-to-prepare, well-balanced daily meals and two healthful snacks that completely satisfy your appetite
- Allows you to vary your calorie intake each weekend and thus avoid feelings of food deprivation and dietary boredom
- Provides you with an easy-to-follow exercise plan that fits in to your daily routine and variations in your schedule
- Changes your body composition so that you become firm, trim, and less flabby
- Changes your body chemistry so that you can more easily manage your weight

IT REALLY WORKS

The New Hilton Head Metabolism Diet not only makes sense, it really works. Over the past ten years, since the original diet has been available to the general public, I have received a flood of letters and telephone calls from successful dieters around the world. Of course, these success stories are too numerous to detail, but I will share with you two recent letters that are typical. The first was from a twenty-nine-year-old woman who had learned of my diet from a good friend of hers who had lost 25 pounds on the Hilton Head plan. The very next day she and her mother bought my book and started dieting. She went on to say, "To my amazement I lost 5 pounds the first week and 4 pounds the second week. I only expected to go back to my old size 12, but I went from 160 pounds (5 feet 5 inches tall), wearing a size 14, to 151 pounds, wearing a size 10." She now weighs 144 pounds and is in a size 8, a size she says she hasn't been able to wear since age ten! She is also delighted by the fact that she has more energy than she's had in years.

The other letter was from a sixty-seven-year-old man who admitted that his wife had been waving my book in his face for several years and he had done his best to ignore her. He eventually relented and set a goal for himself to lose 40 pounds. He achieved his goal twelve weeks later and wrote that his waist size dropped from 46 inches to 38 and that his blood pressure was down to textbook numbers for his age. He added, "There is no way I can ever let myself get overweight again, as long as I have your metabolism diet book. Actually, it's hard to call it a diet since I was never really overly hungry at any time."

I also see the diet work almost every day with clients at my Hilton Head Health Institute. In fact, an independent study conducted by the University of South Carolina showed that almost 70 percent of our clients were still maintaining their weight losses at long-term follow-up contacts.

The statistics surrounding cholesterol reduction on the diet are equally impressive. A recent study of our clients, published in the scientific journal *The Bariatrician*, found an average drop of 34 mg in total cholesterol after only two weeks on the diet.

These results prove that the New Hilton Head Metabolism Diet is no fly-by-night, fad program. It is based on sound theories and has been tested for many years on people just like you. Many of these people had given up on ever being able to manage their weight. It worked for them, and it can work for you too.

Chapter 2

◙ ◙ ◙

THE MYSTERY OF METABOLISM

T he first widespread notion I attacked in developing my plan was that people are overweight because they eat too much. This idea is at the very heart of every diet available. So-called experts think that fat people eat too much because of gluttony, emotional problems, oral needs, or lack of willpower. To this I say, "Nonsense!"

My first rule for you to remember is:

> FAT PEOPLE DO NOT
> EAT MORE THAN
> SLIM PEOPLE

I don't make this statement lightly. An overwhelming number of recent studies support my view. Of course, you might eat ravenously some of the time, but so do slim people. The number of calories you eat cannot account for the difference between your weight and that of a slim friend.

If overeating were the major problem then, other factors being equal, two people eating the same low-calorie diet should lose about the same amount of weight. But, your own experience tells you, this just doesn't happen. Several months ago I saw two nearly identical patients. Both women were in their thirties, five feet five inches tall, and weighed 140 pounds. Neither exercised, and both were very inactive. On a 700-calorie-a-day diet, one lost 6 pounds in three weeks, while the other lost 14 pounds. Both were in a controlled residential program in which dietary meals were carefully portioned out and cheating was not possible. Based on standard notions of overeating as a cause of obesity, these women should have lost the same amount of weight.

Individual differences also show up in nutritional research on overeating. In several studies people have been asked to eat two to three times their usual amount of food to see what happens to their weight. Overweight people who do this gain weight very quickly—as much as 20 pounds in two weeks. Normal-weight and slim people rarely gain more than 5 or 6 pounds.

Well, if overeating is not the problem, then what is? I can answer that in one word—*metabolism*.

THE MISSING LINK: METABOLISM

To understand metabolism, think of your body as a furnace. Food is the fuel that supplies energy to run the furnace. The amount of energy in the food you eat is measured in calories. So you eat calories each day to keep your furnace running. Your furnace burns calories through a process known as metabolism.

Metabolism is simply the energy required to keep you alive. It refers to the number of calories of food energy your body burns to maintain vital functions such as heart rate, brain activity, and digestion. Even if you were in a coma and never moved a muscle, your body would need to burn calories for energy. Generally speaking, metabolism (also known as basal metabolism or resting metabolism) refers to the number of calories your body is burning at rest— when you're not moving or doing anything. Exercise and physical activity also help you burn calories.

All this information can be expressed more simply by means of an energy equation:

$$\begin{array}{ccc} \text{Input} & = & \text{Output} \\ \text{(calories from} & & \text{(calories burned from} \\ \text{food)} & & \text{metabolism} \\ & & \text{and activity)} \end{array}$$

When all the fuel that enters your body is burned up, you maintain your normal weight. Excess fuel that is not burned is stored as fat. If you don't burn all the calories you eat, you will end up with an excess amount of fat.

Since fat people don't eat more than slim people, the cause of overweight must lie in the Output side of the equation. That's exactly right. Fat people do not burn as much fuel (as many calories) as slim people do.

This is my second rule for you to remember:

FAT PEOPLE DO NOT
BURN FAT AS WELL
AS SLIM PEOPLE

Now, you may ask, is this due to problems in metabolism or to a lack of physical activity? It may actually be a combination of both, but it is primarily due to insufficient burning of calories through metabolism. While many overweight people don't get enough exercise, the same can be said of many slim people. There are simply not enough differences in the physical activity levels of fat and slim people to explain weight problems.

METABOLIC SUPPRESSION ·

Before you jump to conclusions, let me assure you that there is nothing abnormal about your metabolism. More than 95 percent of overweight people have a normal thyroid, the gland that controls the number of calories your body burns to keep you alive. Rushing to your doctor to get thyroid supplements won't help. In fact, as I will describe later, taking these hormone supplements when you don't need them will do your metabolism more harm than good.

While your metabolism is not abnormal, it definitely is sluggish and inefficient. You suffer from what I call *metabolic suppression.*

To understand this concept, let's go back to the idea of your body as a furnace. Everyone has a basic, standard level at which he or she burns fuel. This basal metabolism varies from person to person. The average basal metabolism for women is between 1000 and 1500 calories a day—that many calories are burned each day to sustain life. Men have a higher basal metabolism, ranging from 1400 to 1900 calories per day.

In addition to this base level, the rate at which you burn calories fluctuates throughout the day depending on various conditions. For example, your basal metabolism is stimulated when you eat, when the climate changes, and when you exercise. It's like a thermostat automatically turning up the furnace in response to fuel coming in, to any drop in temperature, and to increased energy demand.

If your thermostat is working properly, you have a highly efficient metabolism. Your base rate of, say, 1400 calories will be stimulated several times throughout the day, and you will burn off an extra 400 to 500 calories during each twenty-four-hour period.

People suffering from metabolic suppression often have two problems. First, they are usually at the lower end of the average range of basal metabolism. Second, and even more crucial, their thermostats are defective. Not only do they burn fewer calories, but they do not have the periodic increases in metabolic rate throughout the day. The furnace does not respond to stimulation. Simply, it stays at a low level, regardless of changes in the body or in the environment.

Because of metabolic suppression, a woman could have a base level of only 1100 calories per day and show very slight increases in metabolism—from 50 to 100 calories—during the day. The result could be disastrous. As many as 500 calories of food per day would not be burned off as it should be. That may not seem like a lot, but it adds up to 3500 calories per week, 15,000 calories per month, and 182,500 calories per year. You gain one pound of fat every time your body fails to burn an extra 3500 calories. That means you would gain one pound each week, four or five pounds each month, and more than fifty pounds in a year! A slim person with an efficient metabolism can eat the same number of calories as you and not gain an ounce.

Don't get discouraged. I'm going to show you how to change your metabolism, to fix your thermostat so that you burn more calories. You *can* do it, as long as you follow my plan. Once your body chemistry has been improved, once you release your metabolism to do what it was intended to do, you'll never have a weight problem again. Just think, you'll be like all those slim friends of yours. People will be looking enviously at *you* and saying, "You're one of those naturally slim people. You can eat and not gain weight."

Now that you know what your problem is, you're likely wondering why you have metabolic suppression.

Chapter 3

❋ ❋ ❋

WHY YOUR METABOLISM IS DEFECTIVE

R esearch tells us that the reasons why you gain weight more easily than others is very complex, probably more complex than we ever realized before. Based on our current knowledge, your metabolism may be defective for the following reasons.

1. WHAT YOU INHERITED FROM YOUR RELATIVES: THE "FAT" GENE

We know for sure that certain genetic factors determine whether you will be more prone to fatness than someone else. Just as a tendency to develop high blood pressure or diabetes runs in families, so does the chance of becoming overweight.

If neither of your parents is overweight, you stand about a 20 to 25 percent chance of becoming an overweight adult. If one parent is overweight, your chances double to 40 percent. If your mother *and* father are too heavy, there is an 80 percent chance that you will be, too.

More evidence on this hereditary link comes from studies of twins. Identical twins who have been adopted by different parents and raised apart from each other are a good test of whether biology or environment is more important in determining body weight. When these children with the same genetic makeup but different family settings grow up, they tend to weigh about the same as each other. Furthermore, their body weights correspond more to those of their biological parents than to their adoptive parents.

In 1993, researchers at Rockerfeller University in New York discovered a genetic mutation in obese mice that interferes with proper metabolism and keeps the brain from knowing when to send the signal to stop eating. Although the media headlines declared the discovery of the obesity or "fat" gene with a possible "cure" just around the corner, nothing could be further from the truth.

First, whether this gene works the same way in humans as in mice has yet to be proved. The practical application of this will take years and years of research. Second, the genetics of obesity is a complicated one because the transmission appears to be of a polygenic nature. *Polygenic* refers to the fact that a characteristic (such as being overweight) is linked to more than one gene, whereas a *monogenic* trait is linked to only one gene. The unraveling of the mystery of metabolism and overweight will require the discovery of several genes and how they interact to cause this problem. Unfortunately, there is no one fat gene that will lead to a cure.

Another important factor has to do with "critical stages" of fat-cell development. Given the tendency to be overweight, your eating habits during certain critical times in your life may be more important than how much you eat at other times. Overeating especially in infancy and in adolescence leads to an increase in the number of fat cells in your body—*fat cells that will always be with you*. In addition, women develop more fat cells during pregnancy, which may be why so many trace the history of their weight problems to their childbearing years.

The number of fat cells in your body is important because the more fat cells you have, the greater your chances of gaining weight. Normally, when you gain weight your fat cells get bigger in size, and when you lose weight they get smaller. Unless you are in one of the "critical stages" (infancy, adolescence, or pregnancy), you will not develop any additional fat cells. However, the more fat cells you have, the more will be able to get bigger if you eat too much.

Please don't take all this to mean that if your parents were fat you will automatically be fat and there is nothing you can do about it. I am just presenting the facts and giving reasons why you have more trouble with your weight than some other people do.

In spite of your heredity, you *can* manage and control this "disease." I can't promise that you'll ever be like the person who eats anything and never gains weight. But you can be successful as long as you follow my program. We can tune your metabolic engine so that it works more efficiently.

2. WHO AND WHAT YOU ARE

Other factors such as gender and body size are also important. For example, women have a lower metabolism than men. People who are smaller in height and stature have a lower metabolic rate than taller, larger people. I'll go into more detail on these factors later, but for now just realize that your metabolism may be the way it is because of how tall you are or whether you are male or female. This doesn't mean that your metabolism can't be changed. It simply demonstrates the need for getting on my program to change it.

3. How Often You Diet

It seems strange to suggest that dieting can make your metabolism sluggish, but it's true. Whenever you reduce the number of calories you eat, your body begins to turn down its furnace. The fewer the calories, the lower your metabolism. Your metabolic rate is reduced the most when you suddenly go on a very low-calorie diet or when you fast. Your body is actually fighting the weight loss process by burning fewer calories.

Why? The answer is quite simple. Our bodies are highly adaptive to change and are programmed not for dieting but for survival. When you eat very little or stop eating altogether, your body thinks you are starving. In terms of survival, starvation can eventually lead to death. So your body concludes: "In order to save my life I must conserve energy by burning as few calories as possible." To make matters worse, people who have a low metabolism to begin with show the biggest drop in metabolic rate during dieting.

4. How Much Fat You Eat and How You Diet

The amount of fat in your diet is very much related to weight gain. It's not just how many calories you eat but how fatty those calories are. Your body turns fatty foods into body fat much faster than do other types of foods. So if you eat a lot of fried foods, fatty sauces, high-fat meats, chocolate, butter or margarine, or even salad dressing, you will see the effects on your body very quickly.

Once you have lost weight and are trying to maintain it, you *must* stay on a low-fat diet. Why? Because as an overweight person or even a formerly overweight person, you have a suppressed ability to oxidize, or burn, fat. When you overeat fatty foods, it will affect your weight much more than it would someone who has never had a weight problem.

Inconsistent eating and dieting habits also contribute to metabolic suppression. If you don't eat breakfast, or if you skip meals to lose weight, you are causing your metabolism to become more stingy about burning calories. You are working against yourself.

The very worst pattern of all is one in which periods of dieting are followed by episodes of overeating or bingeing. Unfortunately, this is exactly what happens with most dieters. They go on a very strict diet for several days, eating as little as possible. Then they simply can't stand the deprivation anymore, so they gorge themselves for several days. Once the guilt, depression, and pounds set in, they starve themselves all over again. Sound familiar?

After many repetitions of this pattern the metabolism becomes confused. It declines with dieting and then is expected to bounce right back up quickly when you start eating again. Well, it doesn't. Instead, it rebels. It becomes sluggish and refuses to shoot back up after dieting. It stays suppressed for a much longer time, even after you've stopped dieting. As a result, when you go off your diet your metabolism is still burning very few calories. The food you eat is rapidly turned into fat. In fact, the repetition of this dieting-eating-dieting pattern over the years practically guarantees additional weight gain. If you were trying to get fat and stay that way, you couldn't have chosen a better method.

5. The Diets You Have Tried

Unfortunately, most of the popular diets in the last ten years not only don't help your metabolism but actually contribute to its suppression. The diets that have the worst effect are the following:

- Low-carbohydrate diets
- Fasts
- Liquid diets
- Protein formula diets

Let's suppose you want to lose twenty pounds. You go on one of the many popular low-carbohydrate diets. Now, your body must have a sufficient amount of carbohydrates, primarily in the form of fruits, vegetables, cereal, bread, and potatoes, to supply glucose to the cells. Your cells need glucose for energy. If you're not eating enough carbohydrates to meet your glucose requirements, your body does a very logical thing. It converts the protein you eat into carbohydrate and then into glucose. That's right. Your body has the capability of turning some nutrients into other ones. It's as though your furnace were changing coal into oil.

Now, when that happens—and it happens on *every* diet I've listed—you run into another problem. Since the protein you eat is being changed to carbohydrate, your body doesn't get enough protein to satisfy its protein needs. In its search to fill this need, your body turns to the most readily available alternate source of protein—muscle tissue. It simply burns muscle—your muscle—to provide the missing protein.

In the final analysis you wind up with the following weight loss:

Water loss	=	5	pounds
Fat loss	=	10	pounds
Muscle loss	=	5	pounds

Now, you feel great because you've lost twenty pounds. If only you could look inside your body. It wasn't twenty pounds of fat you lost, only ten. "So what?" you may ask. "Twenty pounds is twenty pounds."

The problem arises when you get off the diet and begin to gain back those pounds. Once you gain back your weight, as most dieters do, the twenty pounds looks like this:

Water gain	=	5	pounds
Fat gain	=	15	pounds
Muscle gain	=	0	pounds

There's your twenty pounds, all right. But look closely. That's not the same twenty pounds you started out with. The low-carbohydrate diet changed your body composition. Somewhere in the process you lost five pounds of muscle and gained five pounds of fat. You're still twenty pounds overweight, but now you are *fatter* than before.

Metabolism is greatly influenced by the ratio of fat to muscle in your body. The more fat and the less muscle, the lower your metabolism. You ended up with a more sluggish metabolism after the diet *because* of the diet. If you had gone on the right kind of dietary program, such as the one I will put you on, this never would have happened. The more fad diets you've been on, the more you've suppressed your metabolism and the more you need my plan.

5. How Active You Are

If you avoid physical activity, your metabolic rate is probably very sluggish. The right kinds of exercise stimulate your metabolism and help you burn more calories. You not only burn calories during physical activity, but for several hours afterward your metabolism remains stimulated. When you've had a very physically active day, you actually end up with a higher metabolic rate that night while you are sleeping because of your exercise. In addition, exercise builds muscle tissue, which changes body chemistry to boost metabolism even higher.

You don't have to become a marathon runner or super athlete to accomplish these goals. I will put you on a reasonable, easy-to-follow physical activity plan that you will enjoy.

ARE YOU A VICTIM OF METABOLIC SUPPRESSION?

If you have doubts about your metabolism, I have developed the following test for you to take. Just answer Yes or No to each question.

METABOLIC SUPPRESSION TEST

	YES	NO
1. Have you had a weight problem off and on for at least two years?	_____	_____
2. Do you frequently skip meals, especially breakfast?	_____	_____
3. Do you fluctuate between periods of dieting and periods of eating too much?	_____	_____

4. Have you been on any liquid
   protein diet, low-carbohydrate diet,
   or very low-calorie diet (fewer
   than 800 calories) more than twice
   in the last few years?   _____   _____

5. When not dieting do you eat a lot
   of high-fat foods?   _____   _____

6. Do you get little or no exercise?   _____   _____

7. Did either of your parents ever
   have a weight problem?   _____   _____

8. Are you female?   _____   _____

9. Are you shorter than 5 feet 5
   inches tall if you are a woman or
   shorter than 5 feet 9 inches tall if
   you are a man?   _____   _____

10. Do you have a history of
    unsuccessful dieting?   _____   _____

Give yourself 10 points for each Yes answer and rate yourself on the scale below:

Score	Metabolic Suppression
0 to 20	None
30 to 40	Mild
50 to 60	Moderate
60 to 70	Severe

Questions and Answers

Q. *What medical tests can I take to see if I have metabolic suppression?*

A. Metabolic suppression, as I have described it, is impossible to detect using standard clinical tests. Your doctor measures your metabolism through a blood test from which he or she determines the amount of thyroid hormone in the bloodstream. These hormones influence the rate of basal metabolism. The results simply tell you if your hormones are within a normal range. A thyroid test cannot tell you how many calories you burn each day.

The exact number of calories you burn can be determined by measuring your oxygen consumption and carbon dioxide output. Unfortunately, the equipment needed to make these determinations is available only at very specialized clinics or at departments of exercise physiology in universities. Additionally, while this equipment could measure your resting metabolic rate, it can't provide an exact determination of the efficiency of your metabolism. (*Efficiency* refers to the ups and downs in your metabolic rate throughout the day.)

Q. *Why has my doctor told me that there is nothing wrong with my metabolism?*

A. Because your test results probably indicate that there is nothing *abnormal* about your thyroid gland. Your doctor has no method of measuring the efficiency of your metabolism.

Q. *If something is wrong with my metabolism, shouldn't I be taking thyroid hormones?*

A. Thyroid supplements are needed by only a very small percentage of people, those who suffer from a glandular abnormality. Metabolic suppression does *not* require thyroid medication. These hormones have little effect if you don't need them. In fact, in the long run, your thyroid gland may react by doing less work.

Q. *If my metabolism is sluggish, will my heart rate and blood pressure be low?*

A. While there is a general relationship between heart rate and metabolism, heart rate is not a reliable indicator of metabolic rate. Blood pressure and metabolism are not related to each other.

Q. *My husband is a very nervous person. Does that mean he has a high metabolism?*

A. Not necessarily. Some people who are nervous have a high metabolism, and some have a low metabolism.

Q. *Which diets should I avoid to keep my metabolism healthy?*

A. Just about all those that have been popular over the past ten years. You should especially avoid diets that are low in carbohydrates, very high in protein, or high in fat. Fasting, liquid diets, and diets below 800 calories should be avoided.

Q. *Why hasn't someone told me all this before?*

A. Because even health professionals know very little about metabolism. Most of the best research in this area is done by a handful of scientists who study metabolism but don't treat overweight patients.

Chapter 4
◼ ◼ ◼
AGE, SEX, AND MUSCLE

Y ou might be wondering what age, sex, and muscle have in common. They all exert a strong influence on metabolic rate. Before I put you on the New Hilton Head Metabolism Diet, you must examine the question, "What makes one person's metabolism different from another's?" You might be amazed to discover that such things as how much muscle you have, what medicines you take, what kind of climate you live in, and how active you are after each meal all affect the number of calories you burn each day.

Following is an outline of the most important influences on your metabolism.

Personal Characteristics

1. Body size
2. Age
3. Sex
4. Muscle-to-fat ratio

BODY SIZE

Generally speaking, the bigger you are, the more calories you burn. It simply takes more energy to run a large furnace than a small one. Your total body size, known scientifically as your "surface area," is based on both your height and weight.

I'll give you an example of the actual difference body size can make. Two of my patients, Barbara and Claire, are both in their midthirties. Both have successfully lost weight and are maintaining their losses. Barbara is small in stature, at five feet one inch and 110 pounds. Claire is a tall woman of five feet nine inches, weighing 140 pounds (an ideal weight for her height). Because of the size difference, Barbara's basal metabolism is 1250 calories per day, while Claire's is 1500. Claire's body burn 250 more calories of energy each day just because she is bigger. This also means that, other factors being equal, Claire can eat 250 calories more than Barbara every day without gaining weight. It may not seem fair, but it's a basic rule of metabolism. The only exception to this rule is in the case of young children. Even though children are much smaller than adults, they burn calories at a much higher rate. This continues until late adolescence. The reason for this higher metabolism is that the bodily processes involved in growth require a great deal of energy. When growth rate declines, so does metabolism.

All this just goes to show you that the determination of metabolism is a very individual matter. The New Hilton Head Metabolism Diet will allow you to take these individual differences into account and use them to your advantage.

AGE

We're all familiar with "middle-age spread." Almost everyone has a friend or relative who was thin all his life, only to develop a substantial "spare tire" around the middle after age forty. Perhaps that friend or relative is you.

As most people realize, metabolism slows down with age. During adulthood the body's energy gradually declines. The most noticeable drop occurs during your mid-forties and slowly continues for the rest of your life.

A fifty-five-year-old person burns about 100 to 150 fewer calories per day than a twenty-five-year-old. That can make a difference of ten to fifteen pounds of excess fat per year. Ten pounds a year may not seem like a lot, but over the years it can quickly add up. One day you might look in the mirror for a little physical self-analysis and find you're forty pounds overweight. Well, those forty pounds weren't gained overnight. Because of changes in metabolism with age, they could very well have accumulated without your eating even one calorie more than you did ten years ago. Dr. Jean Mayer, the noted nutritionist, aptly refers to this age-related fat condition as "creeping obesity."

SEX

Before you get too excited about this section, let me explain that here "sex" refers to your gender, not your behavior. Unfortunately, if you are a woman, your body burns 10 to 15 percent fewer calories each day than does a man's body. Given approximately the same body size, the metabolism of a thirty-five-year-old woman is equal to that of a sixty-five-year-old man! That is why the daily basal metabolism for men ranges between 1400 and 1900 calories, while the basal energy output for women is only 1000 to 1500 calories.

Because of this, men can generally eat more than

women can. They also lose weight more quickly when dieting. Women should never compare their eating patterns or weight losses with those of men. It's like comparing apples and oranges and is a very unrealistic way of looking at weight control.

Please don't get discouraged by these gender differences. They are due mostly to differences in muscle tissue between men and women. By following my system, women can compensate for a large portion of this factor.

MUSCLE

Your body is composed of many different elements and structures, including muscle, fat, skin, bone, water, and internal organs, just to name a few. In terms of metabolism, the most essential ingredients in your body are the amounts of muscle and fat tissue you have.

Let's talk about fat for a minute. You are *supposed* to have fat in your body. Fat is an excellent energy source and a great insulator. It's just that most people have too much fat. Ideally, men should have 15 to 18 percent body fat. Women are by nature supposed to have more fat than men—between 20 and 25 percent is considered ideal. This means that if a woman weighs 135 pounds, approximately 20 percent of her weight—27 pounds—should be composed of fat. With that amount of body fat, a woman would look slim. Unfortunately, most women have a lot more than 20 percent body fat. In fact, the average American woman has about 35 to 40 percent fat. When you are overweight, your body may contain as much as 50 to 60 percent fat. It may seem hard to believe that over half of your total weight on the scale is made up of fat.

Your total weight minus your fat weight is called your "lean body mass." Someone with little fat and a lot of muscle, such as a professional athlete, would have a high lean body mass.

If you weigh 150 pounds and your fat content is 30 percent, your body contains 45 pounds of fat. By subtracting 45 pounds from your weight of 150 pounds, we find that your lean body mass is 105 pounds. You are 45 pounds of fat and 105 of muscle, bone, and everything else.

Why is lean body mass so important? Because one of the most important facts about metabolism is that *the more muscle and the less fat you have, the higher your metabolism is.* People who have a lot of lean body mass burn many more calories per day than do people who have a small amount of lean body mass.

The reason for this is that muscle tissue is metabolically more active than fat tissue. It takes more body energy for muscle to function. Fat is relatively inactive, while muscle cells are extremely active even when you are resting. A muscular furnace is constantly burning food fuel at a rapid rate day after day.

This relationship between lean body mass and metabolism is extremely important. For one thing, it explains why women have a lower metabolism than men. The main reason is that women biologically have more body fat and less muscle than men. When we compare men and women who have similar fat and muscle contents, their metabolic rates are the same. That's great news for women! Your lower metabolism is not inevitable. Women should have a slightly higher fat content than men, but they can close the metabolic gap by achieving their lowest ideal fat percentage. This can be accomplished most effectively through the diet and exercise program of the New Hilton Head Metabolism Diet.

The explanation of why metabolism declines with age is the same. As people get older, their body fat increases. This seems due to the fact that as people age they become less and less physically active. If body fat and muscle tissue remain stable, there is no metabolic decline with age.

Chapter 5

▧ ▧ ▧

MORE QUESTIONS AND ANSWERS ABOUT METABOLISM

Following are some of the most typical questions patients ask me about metabolism.

Q. *When you say I have to reduce my body fat, do you mean that I should have fewer fat cells?*

A. No. As you lose weight, the fat cells you have will shrink in size. You cannot diminish the number of these cells, only their size. The number, in fact, may be genetically determined or may be determined by a combination of heredity and eating patterns in infancy. According to the "fat-cell theory," some people may be born with more fat cells than others and, because of this, gain weight more easily.

Q. *I'd like to stimulate my metabolism by developing more lean body mass, but I don't want to be overly muscular or musclebound.*

A. Don't worry. I don't want you to be overly muscular either. The kind of exercises I prescribe will firm and tone your muscles. You will look slim, trim, and lean, not musclebound.

Q. *I've recently read about brown fat and metabolism in a magazine article. What is brown fat and how does it affect me?*

A. Brown fat (brown adipose tissue) is a special type of fat tissue located in the upper neck and back area. This tissue is found in greatest abundance in newborn infants, small mammals living in cold climates, and animals that hibernate. Some scientists believe this tissue helps to regulate metabolism. They theorize that biochemical activity in this tissue decreases metabolic rate to help animals survive during long periods of hibernation. Recent studies indicate the significance of brown fat in human metabolism is probably minimal.

Q. *I've been taking HCG injections to lose weight. Do these injections stimulate my metabolism?*

A. Definitely not. HCG injections are one of the biggest hoaxes in the treatment of weight control. HCG stands for human chorionic gonadotropin, a hormone found in the urine of pregnant women. These injections were originally developed by two British physicians in Italy and are supposed to help your body burn fat at a faster rate. Every study of these injections has found them to be completely worthless for weight control. They have no effect on your metabolism. The 500-calorie diet that accompanies the injections may actually worsen your metabolic suppression problem.

Q. *I've heard that muscle weighs more than fat. If I lose fat but gain muscle tissue, won't I be defeating my purpose?*

A. No. Although muscle does weigh more than fat, you must decrease fat and increase muscle to speed up your metabolism. You will still lose weight. In fact, you'll also look more trim and compact.

Chapter 6
◪ ◪ ◪
SETTING A REALISTIC WEIGHT GOAL: BODY MASS INDEX AND THE 10 PERCENT SOLUTION

Before you begin the New Hilton Head Metabolism Diet you should figure out how much weight you need to lose. On previous diets you may have used an insurance-company chart to determine your ideal weight. However, experts in the weight control field do not use insurance tables to define overweight. These charts are limited in their usefulness and can be misleading.

The best way for you to find out how overweight you are is by using a measure known as the Body Mass Index (usually referred to as BMI). Rather than compare your weight to some insurance company's standard desirable weight, this measure takes into account the *ratio* between your height and weight.

To obtain this ratio, divide your weight by the square of your height as expressed by the following formula.

$$\text{Body Mass Index} = \frac{\text{Body Weight in Kilograms}}{\text{Height in Meters}}$$

If you're not mathematically inclined, don't panic. I have figured all this out for you. All you have to do is refer to table 1, page 34. I have expressed your weight and height in pounds and inches rather than kilograms and meters.

As you look at table 1, find your height in inches under the Height column. Next, look across the row cor-

TABLE 1

BODY MASS INDEX

HEIGHT	19	20	21	22	23	24	25	26	27	28	29	30	35	40
						Weight								
58"	91	96	100	105	110	115	119	124	129	134	138	143	167	191
59	94	99	104	109	114	119	124	128	133	138	143	148	173	198
60	97	102	107	112	118	123	128	133	138	143	148	153	179	204
61	100	106	111	116	122	127	132	137	143	148	153	158	185	211
62	104	109	115	120	126	131	136	142	147	153	158	164	191	218
63	107	113	118	124	130	135	141	146	152	158	163	169	197	225
64	110	116	122	128	134	140	145	151	157	163	169	174	204	232
65	114	120	126	132	138	144	150	156	162	168	174	180	210	240
66	118	124	130	136	142	148	155	161	167	173	179	186	216	247
67	121	127	134	140	146	153	159	166	172	178	185	191	223	255
68	125	131	138	144	151	158	164	171	177	184	190	197	230	262
69	128	135	142	149	155	162	169	176	182	189	196	203	236	270
70	132	139	146	153	160	167	174	181	188	195	202	207	243	278
71	136	143	150	157	165	172	179	186	193	200	208	215	250	286
72	140	147	154	162	169	177	184	191	199	206	213	221	258	294
73	144	151	159	166	174	182	189	197	204	212	219	227	265	302
74	148	155	163	171	179	186	194	202	210	218	225	233	272	311
75	152	160	168	176	184	192	200	208	216	224	232	240	279	319
76	156	164	172	180	189	197	205	213	221	230	238	246	287	328

responding to your height and find your current weight in pounds. Now follow that column up to the top row of numbers corresponding to your Body Mass Index (ranging from 19 to 40).

The following shows you how to interpret your results.

If your BMI is:	You are:
Higher than 30	Obese
Between 25 and 30	Overweight
Below 25	Healthy weight

You should use your Body Mass Index as a general guideline. For example, if you are in the lower end of the overweight category, with an index of 26 or 27, but are in good health, your present weight may be okay for you. Most experts, however, feel that you should lose weight if your Body Mass Index is higher than 27.

If you have a very high BMI, concentrate on getting it down below 27. If you are in the overweight category, you should set your sights on a BMI below 25.

Keep in mind that BMI is a measure that is correlated with medical health measures. While health may be motivating you to lose weight, you may also be concerned about your appearance. There is no chart that can tell you what is your best weight in terms of how you look and feel. That is completely up to you. For example, if the BMI chart tells you that you would be healthy at a weight of 148, you may still want to weigh less for appearance's sake. This is perfectly okay as long as you don't take it to extremes.

Just remember that you don't *have to* weigh less. You may like the way you look at 135 pounds, but if you find it extremely difficult to maintain that weight, it might not be worth the continual effort it takes. To maintain a weight of 148 pounds may be more realistic because it requires much less exercise and dietary control to maintain. Besides, if you diet *and* follow the exercise program I advise, you will trim up so much that you'll look at least 5 pounds less than you actually weigh.

One final point about your weight goal is that not only should it be realistic but it should be yours. Don't let anyone else choose a goal weight for you. Some of the people who enroll in my institute make this mistake, and we have to persuade them to set their own goals. One fifty-three-year-old woman came to my program to lose 45 pounds because her husband wanted her to look like she had when he married her at age twenty-three. By the way, he weighed 20 pounds more than he had in his twenties, but he saw no need to change himself. After she arrived at the institute this woman changed her goal to a more realistic one and ended up losing 30 pounds. She now looks and feels better and is satisfied with herself as a slimmer fifty-three-year-old. Her husband came to realize that he was being unrealistic, and upon her return home he joined his wife on the New Hilton Head Metabolism Diet and lost 15 pounds.

Your Initial Goal: The 10 Percent Solution

When you begin the New Hilton Head Metabolism Diet, you should set your sights on losing 10 percent of your total body weight, especially if you are very overweight. Remember, this is 10 percent of your total body weight, not 10 percent of the weight you need to lose. Medical research indicates that this "magic" 10 percent is an amount of weight loss that will do wonders for your health and happiness. In fact, if everybody in the United States lost just 10 percent of their body weight, 90 percent of them would show significant improvements in cardiovascular conditions, diabetes, hypertension, and high cholesterol. It seems that we benefit the most from the first few pounds we lose.

If a forty-five-year-old woman is 5'3" tall and weighs 163 pounds, her initial 10 percent goal should be 16 pounds, for a new weight of 147 pounds. Even if she didn't lose any more, and stayed a bit overweight, she would have reduced her BMI from 29 to 26 and have fewer medical problems than if she hadn't lost any weight at all. She would be a lot happier with herself and less likely to struggle with trying to keep off a greater amount of weight.

Once you lose 10 percent, you can set your sights on the next 5 percent or 10 percent using my Dietary Stairstepping approach, which I'll describe later.

A FINAL WORD:
HOW OFTEN YOU SHOULD WEIGH YOURSELF

Before you get started on the New Hilton Head Metabolism Diet, weigh yourself on a reliable scale. If you have an old scale that never seems accurate, buy a new one. Tape a piece of graph paper on the inside of your bathroom door and, every time you weigh, write down the date and your weight.

My rules about weighing:

1. Weigh yourself as soon as you get up on the first day of the diet.
2. After the first weigh-in, weigh yourself once a week and once a week only.

3. Always weigh yourself before breakfast and on the same day of each week.
4. Always weigh yourself undressed or while wearing only light underclothing.

You must resist the urge to weigh yourself every day during the diet. If you are "addicted" to the scale you must avoid weighing yourself several times a day. When you focus your attention on your eating and exercise habits, your weight will take care of itself. Remember, by following my plan you are doing everything you can to speed up your metabolism and lose weight. Your body will lose at its own rate, and there is nothing more you can do.

Some weeks you will lose more than others, regardless of effort. You must look at your weight loss over time and not day to day. When your fat cells lose some of their fat, the void is temporarily filled with water, which may mask your true weight loss for a few days. To weigh daily may be discouraging because you are not getting an accurate picture of what's going on in your body. The scale measures only total body weight at that moment. It doesn't tell you a thing about fat, water, or muscle content in your body.

My parting rule about weighing:

HIDE YOUR SCALE IF YOU MUST,
BUT WEIGH ONLY ONCE A WEEK

Chapter 7
N N N
THE 4 KEY INGREDIENTS TO
REBUILDING YOUR METABOLISM

There are four absolutely essential ingredients to rebuilding your metabolism through dieting. These keys serve as the foundation of the New Hilton Head Metabolism Diet.

KEY INGREDIENT 1:
LOW-FAT FUEL FOR YOUR METABOLISM

The types of foods you eat can help or hinder your body's metabolism. Metabolism is simply the production of heat energy by your body. This internal furnace must be able to regulate itself, to respond to changes just like the furnace in your home does. When you put the wrong kind of fuel in your furnace by eating a poor nutritional diet, you gradually change your body chemistry so that energy output is reduced.

The three basic kinds of fuel that keep your furnace running are protein, carbohydrates, and fats. In fact, these are the only things you eat that your body can burn for energy.

Protein is essential for building and repairing body tissue. It is found in abundance in such foods as chicken, beef, fish, eggs, milk, cheese, lentils, beans, and nuts.

Carbohydrates are sources of long-term energy. There are two basic types: complex and simple. Complex carbo-hydrates are found in fruits, vegetables, potatoes, pasta, cereals, and bread. Simple carbohydrates are sugars such as those found in candy, cookies, ice cream, and soft drinks.

Fat is needed for quick energy and lubrication. Saturated fats (the bad ones, which raise cholesterol) are found in highest concentrations in red meat (white meats have much less), butter, cheese, whole milk, cream, shortening, egg yolks, and palm and coconut oils. Polyunsaturated and monounsaturated fats (the good ones, which may help to lower cholesterol) are found in oils such as safflower, corn, soybean, cottonseed, olive, and peanut.

The amount of fat in your diet is very much related to weight gain. It's not just how many calories you eat but how fatty those calories are. Your body turns fatty foods into body fat much faster than do other types of foods. So if you eat a lot of fried foods, fatty sauces, high-fat meats, chocolate, butter, margarine, or even salad dressing, you will see the effects on your body very quickly.

Once you have lost weight and are trying to maintain it, you must stay on a *very* low-fat diet. Why? *Because as an overweight or a formerly overweight person, you have a suppressed ability to burn fat, especially when you eat a moderate-to-high-fat diet.* When you overeat fats, it will affect your weight much more than would be the case with someone who has never had a weight problem. Unfortunately, this is one of the symptoms of metabolic suppression.

Therefore, the *best* foods to boost your metabolism are:

- Very, very low in fat
- Very high in complex carbohydrates
- Moderate in protein

Years ago, most diets were high in protein and low in carbohydrates. Now we know that eating complex carbohydrates causes you to lose a maximum amount of body fat and a minimum amount of lean body tissue. As we discussed in chapter 2, when your body doesn't get enough dietary carbohydrate, it converts protein into carbohydrate, resulting in protein deficiency. That's when you start burning muscle instead of fat. This is the *worst* thing that can happen to your metabolism. Don't forget—the less muscle, the slower the metabolism.

A diet high in complex carbohydrates and low in fat also helps guard against the drastic declines in metabolism that occur with traditional diets. When you lower your caloric intake on any diet, your metabolism temporarily declines. High-carbohydrate diets help to keep your metabolism strong.

The New Hilton Head Metabolism Diet is *very low* in fat (15 to 20 percent), *very high* in complex carbohydrates (60 percent), and *moderate* in protein (about 20 percent). This is the combination of nutrients that rebuilds your metabolism and makes it stronger.

Low-fat diets may not be new to you as far as your overall health is concerned, but they are more important for weight loss and weight maintenance than we ever thought. The fat content of the New Hilton Head Metabolism Diet is much lower than I previously recommended, both in the low-calorie stage and during maintenance.

KEY INGREDIENT 2:
DIETARY STAIRSTEPPING

When I say *stairstepping* you might be thinking of a new form of exercise. That's not exactly what I had in mind. What I'm referring to is a new concept in achieving your weight goal that we have been experimenting with at my institute. In fact, researchers at Yale and other universities are looking into what I call Dietary Stairstepping with exciting preliminary results.

Before I explain this concept, let's look at the traditional way of losing weight. In the past, if you wanted to lose weight you would simply go on a diet and stay on that diet until you achieved your goal. This is fine if you have only a few pounds to lose, because you wouldn't be dieting for very long. But, what if you have to lose twenty pounds, thirty, fifty, or more?

Three problems arise when you try to "slide" to your goal in this way. First, it is extremely difficult to stick to a low-calorie diet for week after week and month after month without a break. So you end up fluctuating between periods of dieting and periods of not dieting or even of overeating. This on-again/off-again pattern is discouraging, and after a while you may see yourself as a failure.

Second, even if you lose a lot of weight using this sliding approach, you typically put it back on. The reason for this is that during the diet you did not learn anything about what it takes to maintain your weight. Knowing how to lose weight is one thing but keeping it off is quite another. It takes different habits to maintain weight than it does to lose it.

Third, *staying on a low-calorie diet for a long time is not good for your metabolism.* When you diet, your metabolism is suppressed because your body interprets dieting as starvation and a threat to life. By slowing the metabolic rate, your body is trying to save energy in order to keep you alive. The longer you diet, the more your metabolism is suppressed. We can compensate for some of this effect by the short-term dieting recommended in my Booster Weekend phases, but we can't make up for it when you diet continuously for weeks on end, because by then your metabolism is so slow that you will regain some or all of the weight you lost. Fortunately, we can prevent this from happening with Dietary Stairstepping.

With this system, you divide your weight loss goal into steps or stages. You lose some of your weight, maintain that weight loss for a short period of time, lose more weight, maintain again, and so on. It's very much like walking down stairs one step at a time and pausing briefly after each step to catch your breath.

Let's suppose you weigh 166 pounds and you want to lose 36 pounds. Using Dietary Stairstepping, you would divide your weight loss program into three phases or steps of 12 pounds each. Actually, the steps do not need to be of equal amounts. You could lose 16 pounds to begin with and then 10 pounds and then 10 pounds again. This is completely up to you. You will probably lose the first amount of weight faster than subsequent amounts.

The following illustration shows you how your plan would work.

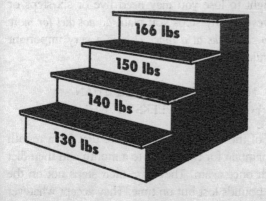

Notice how you lose 16 pounds by going down the first step and then you stop dieting and try to maintain that weight loss for at least two weeks. You then walk down the next step by losing 10 pounds. At that point you stop your low-calorie diet and go to a maintenance plan once again for at least two weeks. Finally, you lose the last 10 pounds and go to permanent maintenance.

At each maintenance step you are rejuvenating your metabolism and preparing it for the next weight loss phase. You are also learning not only how to lose weight but how to keep it off.

I'm sure you have some questions about this method, so I'll go over some of the main issues that people are usually concerned about.

How Much Should I Lose at Each Step?

This is entirely up to you. There is no exact formula. Simply divide your weight into steps, making sure you have a minimum of two or three steps. If you have a great deal of weight to lose you may need five or six steps or more. However many steps you plan, *do not diet for more than four to six weeks at a time*. This is a very important metabolic rule.

NEVER DIET FOR MORE THAN
FOUR TO SIX WEEKS AT A TIME

Many of the clients at my institute diet for a month and then maintain for two weeks to a month and then diet for a month once again. They base their steps not on the number of pounds lost but on time. They accept whatever amount of weight they lose in a month and then try to maintain it until the next step. I like this method because clients worry less about how quickly or how slowly they are losing.

Men lose at a faster rate than women, so they may not need as many steps. A man could lose 25 pounds in two steps while a woman may need three. If you lose weight quickly, your steps can be as short as two weeks in duration.

How Long Should Maintenance Steps Last?

You should maintain your weight between each weight loss step for at least two weeks. It is perfectly okay to maintain for longer periods of time—a month, three months, or even longer.

An Austrian businessman who comes to my program on a yearly basis maintains for eleven months at a time. When he first came to me he had a history of unsuccessful dieting. His busy, hectic lifestyle of international business made it difficult for him to lose weight. He was intrigued by the Dietary Stairstepping approach. He told me he could definitely maintain whatever weight he lost at my institute when he went home but he was not certain he could continue to lose to achieve his final goal.

We set up a plan whereby he enrolls in the institute for one month each year, loses weight on my program, then simply maintains that weight loss for eleven months, until he returns the next year for more weight loss. While most people would not have the patience for this approach, this man did, because as a businessman he had learned the importance of the bottom line—long-term success. Now, after three years he has reached his goal and has been very successful in maintaining it.

Is Dietary Stairstepping for Everyone?

I would strongly encourage everyone to try this approach. It is especially beneficial to someone who has been a yo-yo dieter for years without success. The only people who would not need to use Dietary Stairstepping are those who want to lose only a few pounds.

How Much Should I Eat During the Maintenance Steps?

The number of calories you require to maintain your weight depends on a number of factors including your weight, height, age, gender, and level of exercise. Later in this book, I will provide you with an easy method to calculate your caloric needs at each step of the way.

Are Some People More Successful than Others with This Method?

I believe that everyone who uses this technique will be more successful than those who simply slide to their goal. Everybody who diets is in a hurry to lose weight. They forget that the most important concern is keeping the metabolism strong so that they do not regain the weight they lost. Because of the maintenance steps, Dietary Stairstepping may take a little longer. But by taking these steps you are investing in your future. You are laying a solid foundation so that you will not gain back your weight. What can be more important than that?

This method requires patience, but it also keeps you from becoming bored with continual dieting. Especially if you have a lot of weight to lose, getting a break from low-calorie dieting from time to time keeps you motivated and greatly increases your chances of success.

KEY INGREDIENT 3:
THE THREE-STAGE APPROACH

Ever get bored on a diet, eating the same type and amount of food day after day? Well, most people do. I routinely ask people who have been on other diets, "When you go on a diet, what usually goes wrong? Why can't you stick to it?" Many reply, "I get bored with the same old diet." Others say, "I feel deprived. Everyone else is eating normally and I have to eat diet foods." Or, "I get tired of having to prepare special meals. It takes too much time and effort."

The New Hilton Head Metabolism Diet is definitely different because:

- You will not be bored.
- You will not feel deprived.
- You will not eat "diet" food.

Instead you will be eating normal, everyday foods that everyone else in the family can eat. In addition, the diet includes three stages, and you'll be eating different amounts of food in each stage.

The Weekday Low-Calorie Stage

While some people may be able to lose weight on 1200 or 1500 calories a day, those with metabolic suppression must reduce their intake in the beginning of the diet to 1000 calories a day. Reducing your calories below 1000 per day would be counterproductive since it would not provide your metabolism with the calories needed to keep it strong. On the 1000-calorie level you can and will lose weight. This is the number of calories in my Low-Calorie Stage, which you will follow during the weekdays, Monday through Friday.

The Weekend Booster Stage

The New Hilton Head Metabolism Diet compensates for the fact that your metabolism slows down when you reduce calories. Remember, your body thinks you're starving, so it conserves energy by burning fewer calories. To stir up your metabolism and to keep you from becoming bored with the diet, on the weekends you will switch to the Booster Stage. During this stage you will eat 200 to 250 more calories per day than during the Low-Calorie Stage.

This is like revving up your engine every weekend so that your metabolism doesn't stall out. The switchover to the Weekend Booster Stage is absolutely necessary. It keeps your metabolism strong until we can get you back to a normal number of calories.

The Maintenance Stage

Finally, after you lose each step-determined amount of weight, the Maintenance Stage allows you to keep that weight off. Obviously, this is one of the most important stages, although dieters often forget its importance. They fail to realize that all their effort is wasted if they are unable to keep off their weight. My Maintenance Stage will provide you with just the right formula to maintain your new, lower weight. And, because of my unique Portion Management System, you won't have to worry about counting calories or fat grams.

KEY INGREDIENT 4:
METABOLISM MINIMEALS

How many meals you eat during the day is very important to your metabolism. I'm not talking about how many calories you eat in total, but how they are spaced out.

When dieting, you will lose weight more quickly if you eat several meals a day rather than only one or two meals. Of course, you must eat fewer calories to lose weight, but you will lose it more efficiently if you spread these calories out. How many meals are best? Well, you certainly can't lead a normal life and eat twelve meals a day. It wouldn't be practical, and I'm sure you wouldn't be able to stick to that schedule for very long.

I have found that five meals a day is the optimum number to stir up your metabolism. This number promotes weight loss without interfering with your lifestyle or making you a slave to food. Remember, if you want to keep a strong metabolism, you'll have to continue eating several times a day for the rest of your life. Five low-fat meals a day will keep your weight under control.

The Metabolic Minimeal

You will be eating breakfast, lunch, dinner, plus two metabolic minimeals. These minimeals are really snacks rather than meals. They are simple and require little or no preparation.

The importance of this type of eating pattern was clearly demonstrated by British scientists in a now classic nutritional study. Student volunteers were fed an extra 1800 calories a day for several weeks to see how much weight they would gain. Imagine participating in such a study! Some students were given their 1800 calories all in one meal. Others were given it in small portions throughout the day, about 100 calories each hour. Even though all the students were eating the same number of extra calories, the "one meal" students gained considerably more weight than did those receiving numerous small meals. Somehow, the students who ate small meals were able to burn up more food calories. How was this possible? Actually, the answer is quite simple. It is the result of a common metabolic process that has been recognized since the 1920s.

Dietary Thermogenesis

Without realizing it, these students were experiencing "dietary thermogenesis." This bodily response occurs after every meal or snack you eat. Food entering your body stimulates your metabolism. Whenever you eat, your body burns more calories because of the extra energy needed to digest and absorb the food. Your furnace is charged up to burn the fuel entering your body. It was once thought that only protein foods stimulated the metabolism. We now realize that carbohydrates and fats also have this effect.

Dietary thermogenesis is extremely significant in controlling your weight. *After a meal, your metabolism increases between 10 and 30 percent. It remains stimulated for the next one to three hours.* The more meals you eat, the more your metabolism is stimulated. With a thermogenic response of 20 percent you could be burning an extra 20 calories after each meal. By eating five times a day, you would be burning an extra 100 calories daily without even trying.

Overweight people are at a distinct disadvantage when it comes to dietary thermogenesis. That's because they suffer from metabolic suppression. The average increase in metabolism after a meal is 26 percent for someone who is lean with little body fat. People with too much fat show an increase of only 9 percent and in some cases as low as 3 percent. The problem can be critical since it can account for 70 calories a day that you're not burning properly. This may not seem like a lot, but 70 unburned calories a day over a year translates into a weight gain of *more than seven pounds!*

The moral of this story is that you must eat five times a day—three meals and two healthful snacks. A little later I'll discuss when you should eat these meals and how you should space them out.

Chapter 8

N N N

THE NEW HILTON HEAD
METABOLISM DIET

Now you're ready to begin. Remember, you're not simply going to lose weight on this program. The real goal is to improve your metabolism so that weight loss and maintenance of that weight loss become easier for you.

After several days on the diet you will notice three feelings that may surprise you:

1. You will have very little hunger.
2. You will have loads of energy.
3. You will feel in control of your body.

Many people are sure that they will feel hungry, deprived, and fatigued on a diet. The New Hilton Head Metabolism Diet is so well balanced and has such a positive effect on your metabolism that you will feel energetic and satisfied. After two weeks on the diet, a working mother of two small children said to me, "I have so much energy I can't believe it. I'm able to get twice as much work done and energy to spare. I'm finally finding time to do things for me—to do some of the things I really enjoy. And I'm a lot less cranky at work and at home. I haven't felt hungry once since I started your diet, even though I'm eating so much less than I normally do!"

STAGES OF THE NEW HILTON HEAD METABOLISM DIET

The New Hilton Head Metabolism Diet is different from any diet you've ever been on. Because I am trying to help you change your metabolism, you *must* follow my diet exactly as it is prescribed. Do not make changes on your own.

As mentioned earlier, the New Hilton Head Metabolism Diet has three stages. You must go through all three stages to be successful.

Stage 1: The Weekday Low-Calorie Stage

Begin with the Low-Calorie Menu Plan. This stage is designed for maximum weight loss. *Follow this menu plan during the week from Monday through Friday.*

Stage 2: The Weekend Booster Stage

Every Saturday and Sunday, switch to the Booster Menu Plan. This stage allows a few more calories and is designed to boost your metabolic rate and compensate for your body's "survival response," which I discussed earlier. Even though this stage provides more calories, you will still lose weight. You must switch to the Booster Stage on the weekends to keep your metabolism strong.

Stage 3: The Maintenance Stage

When you reach your weight goal (either your intermediate Dietary Stairstepping goal or your final goal weight), switch to the Maintenance Stage. This plan is designed to boost your metabolism to its maximum level and enable you to maintain your new weight without gaining.

The Metabolic Minimeal

The New Hilton Head Metabolism Diet provides you with five delicious meals every day. You must eat all five meals for the diet to work properly. *Never skip a meal under any circumstances.* Remember, your metabolism increases after every meal, enabling you to burn more calories for the next one to three hours.

In addition to breakfast, lunch, and dinner (or supper, if you prefer), you will be eating two minimeals each day. These minimeals are actually healthful snacks of about 100 calories each. I refer to them as "meals" because I want you to think of them as important and essential to your overall diet. They are not optional. Think of these minimeals as being as important as any other meal of the day.

As you'll see, I have kept these minimeals simple so they don't require a lot of preparation. For example, the easiest minimeal is a piece of fruit that is easy to carry with you if need be.

I suggest you eat one minimeal between lunch and dinner and the other between dinner and bedtime. Make sure you allow at least two hours after your last meal. If you eat breakfast or lunch late on a particular day, it's perfectly okay to have one of your minimeals in the late morning.

Don't be afraid to eat one of your minimeals between dinner and bedtime. You may have been told in the past that you shouldn't eat in the evening or near bedtime. As long as you are spreading out your food intake over the entire day, you don't have to worry. Even if you eat your minimeal an hour before bedtime, it's not a problem. Eating raises your metabolism, as discussed earlier, and that effect doesn't change even if you're lying down or sleeping.

THE 6 BASIC RULES OF
THE NEW HILTON HEAD METABOLISM DIET

Make sure you read all of these rules carefully before beginning the diet.

1. Basic Food Rule

Eat everything exactly as it is prescribed. However, if you are allergic to certain foods or if you have a strong dislike for them, substitutions are provided for you (see chapter 17). Do not eat anything other than what my menu plan recommends. Buy fresh or frozen fruits and vegetables and avoid the canned varieties. Remove all visible fat from meat and remove the skin from chicken before cooking it.

2. Portion-Control Rule

Measure all recommended portions so that you do not eat more than you should. It is common to eat too much unless you measure portions very carefully using measuring cups and a food scale. Before you begin the diet, buy a food scale and a good set of measuring cups. In restaurants or when eating at someone else's home, do the best you can by trying to estimate portions. Measuring food portions will become even more important during the maintenance stage, when you put my Portion Management System into effect.

3. Water Rule

Drink at least five 8-ounce glasses of water or other noncaloric beverages (such as diet soft drinks). Choose noncaloric drinks that are also noncaffeinated. Caffeine is a diuretic and robs your body of fluid. If you must have a cup of caffeinated coffee or tea in the morning to get you going, make sure that is the only caffeine you drink during the day.

4. Salt Rule

Do not add salt to your food while cooking or at the table. You get plenty of sodium naturally in the foods that you eat. Overconsumption of sodium is not healthy especially if you have high blood pressure. Eating salty foods may also cause you to retain fluid, which will mask your true weight loss when you weigh yourself.

5. Alcohol Rule

During the Weekday Low-Calorie and Weekend Booster Stage avoid alcoholic beverages. During the Maintenance Stage you may have alcohol in moderation.

6. Vitamin Rule

It is important to take a multivitamin/mineral supplement each day. Prior to menopause, women should take a supplement that contains iron. Men and postmenopausal women do not require iron. Women should take one to two 500- or 600-mg tablets of calcium per day in the form of calcium carbonate. Multivitamin/mineral and calcium supplements are available at your local pharmacy.

Now let's get started. Following is the Weekday Low-Calorie Menu Plan. Keep in mind that the number of ounces indicated for fish, meat, or chicken refers to *cooked* ounces. You should buy about two ounces more than you need to allow for shrinkage during cooking.

BEFORE WE BEGIN:
A WORD ABOUT CALORIES AND FAT GRAMS

Remember, you don't have to worry about counting calories or fat grams. I have done that for you. There is no need to list calories and fat grams for each day of the menu plan because the New Hilton Head Metabolism Diet has been designed so that each day has approximately the same number of calories and fat grams. There will be some slight variations, but basically *the menu plan provides the following per day:*

- Calories: No more than 1000 per day
- Fat grams: No more than 15 to 20 grams
- Calories from fat: Less than 20 percent

Since I have figured your fat grams and calories, I want you to pay particular attention to *portion sizes*. When you are preparing food at home, **you must measure every portion in the menu plan below using a measuring cup, measuring spoons, or a measuring scale. This is extremely important!**

Weekday Low-Calorie Menu Plan (Monday Through Friday)

The Weekday Low-Calorie Menu Plan includes breakfast, lunch, dinner, and minimeals for Monday through Friday. Remember, minimeals, or snacks, should be eaten about halfway between lunch and dinner and, once again, halfway between dinner and bedtime. Chapter 9 will give you the Weekend Booster Menu Plan for Saturday and Sunday.

Breakfast Every Day

Cereal	3/4 cup of any low-fat (less than 2 grams per serving) high-fiber cereal (cold or hot)
(or)	
Toast	2 slices of low-calorie whole wheat bread or 1 oat bran English muffin with 1 tablespoon of low-sugar jam or jelly
Milk	2/3 cup skim or 1%
Fruit	Choice of 1 whole banana, orange, apple, pear, 1/2 cantaloupe, 1/4 medium honeydew, or any equivalent fruit listed in chapter 17
Beverage	Choice of coffee or tea with sugar substitute and/or a dash of skim or 1% milk, if desired, or water or any other noncaloric beverage

Alternative Breakfasts That You May Choose for Variety *(Once a Week Only!)*

French toast	2 slices of low-calorie bread prepared with 2 egg whites, and 1 tablespoon of commercially prepared low-calorie syrup
Fruit	Choice of 1 whole banana, orange, apple, pear, 1/2 cantaloupe, 1/4 medium honeydew, or any equivalent fruit listed in chapter 17
Beverage	Choice of coffee or tea with sugar substitute and/or a dash of skim or 1% milk, if desired, or water or any other noncaloric beverage

(or)

Egg	1 whole cooked egg, any way you like it. If fried, use vegetable cooking spray; if scrambled, use 1 teaspoon or less of diet margarine
Toast	2 slices of toasted low-calorie whole wheat bread with 1 tablespoon of low sugar jam or jelly, if desired
Orange	1/2
Beverage	Choice of coffee or tea with sugar substitute and/or a dash of skim or 1% milk, if desired, or water or any other noncaloric beverage

*Note: This egg breakfast will add 5 to 6 grams of fat to your daily total. This is not anything to worry about on this low-fat diet *as long as you do not eat this breakfast more than once per week.* You may want to substitute one of the commercially prepared, low-fat, low-cholesterol egg products for the egg.

Lunch and Dinner Menus

MONDAY

Lunch

Tuna salad sandwich	1/4 cup of tuna salad (see recipe on p. 214) on 2 slices of low-calorie whole wheat bread with lettuce and 2 slices of tomato
Carrots	6 raw baby carrots or small carrot sticks

Beverage   Choice of any noncaloric or
                                low-calorie beverage (for
                                example, diet soft drink)

Minimeal
Fruit   Choice of 1 apple, pear,
                                orange, banana, or any
                                equivalent fruit listed in
                                chapter 17

Dinner
Pasta   1 1/4 cups of cooked pasta
                                with 1/2 cup of commercially
                                prepared tomato sauce or 1
                                serving of any of the pasta
                                recipes on pp. 157 to 167
Salad   Small dinner salad with
                                lettuce, tomato, cucumber, and
                                1 tablespoon of low-fat
                                dressing of choice
Beverage   Choice of any noncaloric or
                                low-calorie beverage

Minimeal
Fruit or popcorn   Choice of 1 fruit or 4 cups of
                                air-popped popcorn with no
                                butter or salt

TUESDAY

Lunch
Grilled cheese sandwich   2 slices of low-calorie whole
                                wheat bread with 1 slice of

	low-fat American cheese and 2 slices of tomato, grilled with nonstick vegetable cooking spray
Soup	1 cup of commercially prepared vegetable soup (choose a brand labeling their soup as "light" or "healthier," having no more than 2 grams of fat per serving)
Beverage	Choice of any noncaloric or low-calorie beverage

Minimeal

Fruit	1 whole banana, orange, apple, pear, peach, or any equivalent fruit listed in chapter 17

Dinner

Chicken	3 ounces of baked chicken, sprinkled with any commercially prepared low-sodium spice/seasoning mix or 1 serving of any of the chicken recipes on pp. 170 to 185
Potato	1/2 baked potato with 1 teaspoon of diet margarine
Vegetables	1 cup of cooked carrots, broccoli, green beans, or mixed vegetables
Beverage	Choice of any noncaloric or low-calorie beverage

Minimeal
Fruit	1 whole banana, orange, apple, pear, peach, or any equivalent fruit listed in chapter 17

WEDNESDAY

Lunch
Salad	Mixture of lettuce, onions, tomatoes, mushrooms, green peppers, radishes, and a choice of 1/2 cup of low-fat cottage cheese or 2 ounces of diced chicken served with 3 tablespoons of low-fat, diet dressing of choice. Serve with 3 fat-free crackers or melba toast
Beverage	Choice of any noncaloric or low-calorie beverage

Minimeal
Fruit	1 whole banana, orange, apple, pear, peach, or any equivalent fruit listed in chapter 17

Dinner
Fish	5 ounces of baked fish (any type) with lemon juice or 1 serving of any of the fish recipes on pp. 196 to 207

Potato	1/2 baked potato or 1 serving of Oven Fries (no-fat version of French fries) using recipe on p. 216
Vegetables	1/2 cup of cooked carrots, green beans, broccoli, or any equivalent vegetable listed in chapter 17
Beverage	Choice of any noncaloric or low-calorie beverage

Minimeal

Raw veggies	2 cups of raw vegetables, including (according to choice) baby carrots or small carrot sticks, small celery sticks, broccoli, cauliflower, and/or radishes served with 1/4 cup of commercially prepared low-calorie, low-fat dip, if desired

THURSDAY

Lunch

Potato	1 medium to large baked potato, split open and topped with 1/2 cup of chopped broccoli and 1 slice of melted low-fat American or cheddar cheese
Beverage	Choice of any noncaloric or low-calorie beverage

Minimeal

Fruit

Choice of banana, pear, apple, peach, orange, or any equivalent fruit listed in chapter 17

Dinner

Veal

3 to 4 ounces of cooked veal steak using any of the veal recipes listed on pp. 192 to 195. Portion would be equivalent to 1 serving of Veal Piccata or Veal Parmesan. If you prefer not to eat red meat, substitute chicken for the veal

Rice

1/2 cup of cooked rice, or use any of the recipes for rice on pp. 219 to 222 for variety

Minimeal

Mixed fruit

3/4 cup of chopped, mixed fruit of any variety, or 1 serving of Fruit Ambrosia or Fruit Parfait (see recipes on p. 231)

FRIDAY

Lunch

Stuffed pita bread

1 pita bread stuffed with 2 ounces of chopped chicken, tuna, or turkey, 1/2 tomato diced, 1 cup of chopped

| | lettuce, and 2 tablespoons of fat-free Italian salad dressing |
| Beverage | Choice of any noncaloric or low-calorie beverage |

Minimeal

| Fruit or veggies | 1 whole fruit of your choice or 1 1/2 cups of mixed raw vegetables (carrots, celery, etc.) |

Dinner

Fish or shrimp	5 ounces of fish (any variety) or shrimp with 2 tablespoons of commercially prepared cocktail sauce
Corn	1 medium ear of corn with 1 teaspoon diet margarine
Cole slaw	1/2 cup of cole slaw prepared with nonfat salad dressing or according to recipe on p. 209
Beverage	Choice of any noncaloric or low-calorie beverage

Minimeal

| Fruit | 1 cup of mixed chopped fruit of your choice topped with 1/4 cup of low-fat plain yogurt |

Saturday and Sunday
See chapter 9 for Weekend Booster Menu Plan

MONDAY

Lunch

Chicken sandwich	3 ounces of sliced chicken or turkey with lettuce, 2 slices of tomato, and 1 teaspoon of low-fat mayonnaise served on a whole wheat roll
Fruit with yogurt	1/2 cup of berries, grapes, or diced melon with 2 tablespoons of low-fat plain yogurt

Minimeal

Pretzels	1 ounce (number of pretzels in an ounce varies depending on their size and shape)

Dinner

Stir-fry	1 cup of vegetables (any mix of diced vegetables), 3 ounces of diced pork or chicken, and 1/4 cup of low-sodium teriyaki sauce, prepared by stir-frying
Rice	1/2 cup of brown rice (serve stir-fry over rice)
Beverage	Choice of any noncaloric or low-calorie beverage

Minimeal

Fruit

1 whole apple, orange, banana, pear, peach, or any equivalent fruit listed in chapter 17

TUESDAY

Lunch

Tuna melt sandwich

1/4 cup of tuna salad (mix water-packed tuna with 1 teaspoon of low-fat mayonnaise or see recipe on p. 214), 2 slices of low-calorie whole wheat bread, 1 slice of low-fat cheese melted over tuna salad

Lettuce and tomato

3 slices of tomato on lettuce leaf

Beverage

Choice of any noncaloric or low-calorie beverage

Minimeal

Fruit

1 whole apple, banana, orange, pear, or any equivalent fruit listed in chapter 17

Dinner

Lasagna

1 portion of Lasagna (see recipe on p. 162) or 1 serving of any of the other pasta dishes on pp. 157 to 167

Salad

1 small dinner salad with lettuce, tomato, cucumbers,

	radishes, etc., topped with 1 tablespoon of fat-free dressing
Beverage	Choice of any noncaloric or low-calorie beverage

Minimeal

Sherbet, sorbet, or fruit	1/2 cup of fruit-flavored sherbet/sorbet (with no sugar added) or 1 whole fruit

WEDNESDAY

Lunch

Large chef's salad	In a large salad bowl, mix 2 cups of chopped lettuce, 1/2 tomato diced, 5 slices of cucumber, 3 bell pepper rings, 3 onion rings, 2 ounces diced chicken or turkey, 1 teaspoon of Parmesan cheese, and 2 tablespoons of low-fat Italian dressing
Crackers/melba toast	3 to 4 fat-free crackers or melba toast
Beverage	Choice of any noncaloric or low-calorie beverage

Minimeal

Fruit	1 whole apple, orange, banana, pear, or any equivalent fruit listed in chapter 17

Dinner

Fish	5 ounces of any fish baked with 1 teaspoon of diet margarine and lemon juice or 1 serving of any of the fish recipes on pp. 196 to 207
Potato	1/2 baked potato with 1 teaspoon of diet margarine or 1 serving of Mashed Potatoes or Oven Fries (see recipes on p. 216)
Vegetable	1/2 cup of any of the Group I vegetables listed on p. 154
Beverage	Choice of any noncaloric or low-calorie beverage

Minimeal

Popcorn	4 cups of air-popped popcorn with no butter or salt

THURSDAY

Lunch

Chicken or turkey sandwich	3 ounces of sliced chicken or turkey with lettuce, 2 slices of tomato, and 1 teaspoon of diet mayonnaise served on 2 slices of low-calorie whole wheat bread
Fruit with yogurt	1/2 cup of berries, grapes, or diced melon, with 1 tablespoon of low-fat plain yogurt if desired

Beverage   Choice of any noncaloric or
                            low-calorie beverage

Minimeal

Choose your favorite minimeal from any of the preceding days

Dinner

Macaroni and cheese   1 serving of Macaroni and
                            Cheese (see recipes on pp. 163
                            to 164) or 1 1/4 cups of pasta
                            with 1/2 cup of commercially
                            prepared meatless spaghetti
                            sauce
Broccoli   1 cup of broccoli florets
Beverage   Choice of any noncaloric or
                            low-calorie beverage

Minimeal

Cereal   3/4 cup of any low-fat cereal
Milk   2/3 cup of skim or 1% milk

FRIDAY

Lunch

Primavera salad   2 cups of any pasta/vegetable
                            combination or 1 serving of
                            Pasta Primavera (see recipe on
                            p. 161)
Beverage   Choice of any noncaloric or
                            low-calorie beverage

Minimeal

Fruit | 1 whole apple, banana, orange, pear, or any equivalent fruit listed in chapter 17

Dinner

Hamburger | 2 ounces of ground round broiled and served on a whole wheat hamburger bun with lettuce, sliced tomato, and 1 tablespoon of "light" ketchup (3 ounces of ground turkey may be substituted for the ground round, if desired)

Potato | 1 serving (1/2 potato) of Oven Fries (see recipe on p. 216)

Beverage | Choice of any noncaloric or low-calorie beverage

Minimeal

Fruit | 1 whole apple, banana, orange, pear, or any equivalent fruit listed in chapter 17

WHAT HAPPENS AFTER THIS TWO-WEEK MENU PLAN?

If you are dieting for more than two weeks, simply start over and repeat the menu plan. On weekends you will eat my Booster Menu Plan, described in chapter 9. Remember, with my Dietary Stairstepping technique, you will not stay on the Weekday Low-Calorie Plan for more than six weeks. Then you will need to switch to the Maintenance Stage, described in chapter 10, for at least two weeks before returning to the low-calorie menus.

SUBSTITUTIONS AND VARIATIONS

While you should try to follow these menu plans as closely as possible, I realize that substitutions and variations are necessary from time to time. I have tried to give you enough of a choice within each meal to allow for individual likes and dislikes. For example, for most of the dinner meals I have given you a fairly simple main dish and then offered suggestions from my recipes, in chapter 18, as alternatives.

Depending on your schedule, you may substitute one day's lunch for the lunch on another day. The same is true of the dinners. While I do want you to stick to a dietary plan, you need not be rigid about it.

EASY-TO-FOLLOW MENUS

In looking over the Weekday Low-Calorie Menu Plan, you've probably noticed how practical and easy to follow it is. The meals consist of common, everyday foods that are easy to buy and easy to prepare. No fancy or expensive "diet" foods are included. Plenty of variation in day-to-day meals is provided. You'll be especially thankful for this variety if you've ever been on very restrictive diets such as the liquid protein ones.

One of my clients told me, "Your diet is so easy. It takes very little time to prepare, and I can serve my family the same food—just more of it. I don't have to prepare two separate meals for myself and the family. Even when we eat out, I can order something that's pretty close to your menu plan."

Chapter 9

◪ ◪ ◪

THE WEEKEND BOOSTER STAGE

On Saturdays and Sundays you must switch from the Weekday Low-Calorie Menu Plan to the Weekend Booster Menu Plan. The Booster Stage provides an extra 200 to 250 calories per day more than the Low-Calorie Stage. Do not hesitate to switch to the Booster Stage on the weekends.

Clients say to me, "If I'm losing weight on the low-calorie menus, why eat more calories? Maybe I'd lose even more weight if I ate even fewer calories." Wrong! Wrong! Wrong! This is just the kind of thinking that caused your metabolism problem in the first place.

You *must* switch to the Booster Stage on weekends for my system to work. We must keep jolting your metabolism. Prolonged low-calorie dieting puts your metabolism to sleep, which is just what we're trying to prevent.

You *will* lose weight during the Booster Weekends. You will continue to lose because even though you are eating slightly more, you are also burning more. Your metabolism has speeded up. I assure you, based on my twenty years of experience, that you will keep losing at a good rate.

Keep in mind that my system has been developed carefully and has been tested on thousands of people. It definitely works if you follow my guidelines, but you must make sure to follow every one of them.

*W*eekend Booster Menu Plan
(Saturday and Sunday)

First Weekend

SATURDAY

Breakfast

Same as low-calorie breakfast (including alternatives) described in chapter 8, but *add 6 ounces of fruit juice* (orange, apple, cranberry, or any type you prefer)

Lunch

Tuna or chicken melt	1/2 cup of tuna salad or chicken salad (see recipes on pp. 214 and 208), served open-faced on an oat bran English muffin with 1 slice of low-fat American cheese (broil to melt cheese on top)
Lettuce and tomato	Lettuce leaves topped with 3 slices of tomato
Beverage	Choice of any noncaloric or low-calorie beverage

Minimeal

Fruit	1 whole fruit of your choice

Dinner

Pasta	1 1/4 cups of cooked spaghetti or vermicelli noodles with 1/2 cup of commercially prepared

	tomato sauce or 1 serving of any of the pasta recipes on pp. 157 to 167
Bread or roll	1 slice of Italian bread or 1 dinner roll
Salad	small dinner salad with lettuce, tomato, cucumber, radishes, and 1 tablespoon of fat-free dressing of choice
Beverage	Choice of any noncaloric or low-calorie beverage

Minimeal

Any minimeal from the Weekday Low-Calorie Menu Plan

SUNDAY

If you eat your larger meal in the middle of the day, feel free to exchange the lunch and dinner menus

Breakfast

Same as Weekday Low-Calorie breakfast (including alternatives) described in chapter 8, but *add 6 ounces of fruit juice* (orange, apple, cranberry, or any type you prefer)

Lunch

| Pita pizza or Stuffed baked potato | 1 serving of either Pita Pizza (see recipe on p. 169) or Stuffed Potato (see recipe on p. 219) |
| Salad | small dinner salad with 1 tablespoon low-fat dressing of choice |

Beverage

Choice of any noncaloric or
low-calorie beverage

Minimeal

Fruit

Choice of 1 apple, orange,
banana, pear, or any equivalent
fruit listed in chapter 17

Dinner

Meatloaf

1 serving of Mom's Meatloaf
(see recipe on p. 191) or, as a
substitute, 1 serving of any
other meat recipe on pp. 186
to 195

(If you prefer to avoid red meat, substitute 1 serving
of any chicken recipe on pp. 170 to 185)

Potato

1 serving of Mashed Potatoes
(see recipe on p. 216) or any
other potato recipe on pp. 216
to 219

Vegetable

3/4 cup of cooked carrots,
broccoli, green beans, spinach,
or mixed vegetables

Minimeal

Popcorn or raw veggies

4 cups of air-popped popcorn
without salt or butter or 2
cups of raw vegetables such as
baby carrots or small carrot
sticks, small celery sticks,

radishes, and cauliflower
florets served with 1/4 cup of
commercially prepared low-
calorie, low-fat dip

Second Weekend

SATURDAY

Breakfast

Same as Weekday Low-Calorie breakfast (including alternatives) described in chapter 8, but *add 6 ounces of fruit
juice* (orange, apple, cranberry, or any type you prefer)

Lunch

Fruit Salad	Wedges of 1/2 orange, slices of 1/2 apple, and 1/2 cup of grapes, arranged on lettuce and served with 1/2 cup of low fat cottage cheese
Crackers/melba toast	4 fat-free crackers or melba toast
Beverage	Choice of any noncaloric or low-calorie beverage

Minimeal

Bagel or English muffin	1 bagel (2-ounce variety) or 1 oat bran English muffin with 1 tablespoon of diet margarine or 1 tablespoon of sugar-free jam or jelly

Dinner

Chicken	3 ounces of baked chicken (without skin and seasoned to taste with commercially prepared low-sodium seasoning mix), or 1 serving of any of the chicken recipes on pp. 170 to 185
Rice	3/4 cup of cooked brown rice or 3/4 cup of any of the rice recipes on pp. 219 to 222
Vegetables	1 cup of mixed vegetables (choose your favorites)
Beverage	Choice of any noncaloric or low-calorie beverage

Minimeal

Banana/strawberry surprise	1/2 sliced banana mixed with 1/2 cup of sliced strawberries topped with 1 tablespoon of low-fat plain yogurt

SUNDAY

Breakfast

Same as low-calorie breakfast (including alternatives) described in chapter 8, *but add 6 ounces of fruit juice* (orange, apple, cranberry, or any type you prefer)

Lunch

Macaroni and Cheese	2 servings of Macaroni and Cheese (see recipes on p. 163)
Vegetable	1/2 cup of cooked broccoli

| Beverage | Choice of any noncaloric or low-calorie beverage |

Minimeal

| Fruit | 1 whole apple, orange, banana, pear, or any equivalent fruit listed in chapter 17 |

Dinner

Fish	5 ounces of baked fish (any type) with lemon juice or 1 serving of any of the fish recipes on pp. 196 to 207
Potato or rice	1 whole baked potato or 3/4 cup of rice (use any of the rice recipes on pp. 219 to 222)
Vegetable	1/2 cup of cooked carrots, green beans, broccoli, asparagus, or any equivalent vegetable listed in chapter 17
Beverage	Choice of any noncaloric or low-calorie beverage

Minimeal

| Popcorn | 4 cups of air-popped popcorn with no salt or butter |

If you are staying on the New Hilton Head Metabolism Diet for more than two weeks, simply repeat the Weekday Low-Calorie and Weekend Booster Menu Plans using my recipes in chapter 18 for variety. When you have reached your first goal in Dietary Stairstepping, refer to the following chapter, chapter 10, for my Maintenance Menu Plan.

Chapter 10

◪ ◪ ◪

The Maintenance Stage: Using My Portion Management System to Keep Your Weight Off

As you recall from chapter 7, my Dietary Stairstepping technique requires you to discontinue the Weekday Low-Calorie and Weekend Booster Menu Plans after four to six weeks or after you have lost your first-step goal weight. Then, for at least two weeks, you should enter the Maintenance Stage. Remember, between each step in Dietary Stairstepping you should follow the Maintenance Stage recommendations for two weeks. This stage is also designed for you to follow after you have lost all the weight you choose to lose.

The Maintenance Stage is designed to balance your metabolic energy equation, as we discussed in chapter 2. Because you are trying to maintain rather than lose weight, you will be able to eat many more calories than were prescribed in either the Weekday Low-Calorie or the Weekend Booster Stages. During the Maintenance Stage we must make certain that the number of calories you eat is the same as the number of calories you burn through metabolism and physical activity.

The key to the Maintenance Stage is my *Portion Management System*, which frees you from having to count calories or fat grams. As long as you pay attention to serving sizes of foods you will never have to worry about calories again. To implement this system you must first determine how many calories you should eat to maintain your weight. Then you can use the recommendations of my Portion Management System that correspond to the calorie range you need.

To find out how many calories you should eat to maintain a certain weight, we must return to the energy equation. Remember, your goal in the Maintenance Stage is to ensure that:

$$\text{Caloric Input} = \text{Caloric Output}$$

Determining maintenance calories is quite simple. If you ask, "How many calories should I eat to maintain a weight of 140 pounds?", the answer is simple: "As many as you can burn off." To find your maintenance Input we must first calculate your maintenance Output.

To measure your total output, we must compute your metabolic rate and then add calories you burn through physical activity.

How to Estimate Your Resting Metabolism

There are a number of ways to determine your metabolic rate (some a lot simpler than the one I use), but the following method is very accurate because it takes into account your weight, height, age, and gender. This formula requires several calculations, so get out your calculator and let's get started.

There are different methods for men and women, so be sure you use the one appropriate for your gender.

Metabolism Formula for Women

$$\text{Metabolic Rate} = (\text{Weight Factor} + 655.1) + \text{Height Factor} - \text{Age Factor}$$

Before we work out the answer, we must first calculate the Weight, Height, and Age Factors that go into the formula.

To find your *Weight Factor*

1. Multiply your maintenance weight in pounds by 4.302
2. The answer is your Weight Factor

To find your *Height Factor*

1. Multiply your height in inches by 4.625
2. The answer is your Height Factor

To find your *Age Factor*

1. Multiply your age by 4.68
2. The answer is your Age Factor

Now that we have these three factors, we can go back to the formula and simply fill in the numbers. Here's how to do it:

1. Add 655.1 to your Weight Factor
2. Add your Height Factor to the answer
3. Subtract your Age Factor from that answer
4. Multiply that answer by .85
5. The resulting number is your daily metabolic rate (how many calories you burn without exercise)

Remember, you'll be able to eat more than your resting metabolic rate at the Maintenance Stage because we have not yet added physical activity. We'll do that as soon as I give you the metabolic formula for men. When you have finished your calculations, go directly to the section "Finding Your Total Output by Adding Physical Activity."

Metabolism Formula for Men

$$\text{Metabolic Rate} = (\text{Weight Factor} + 66.5) + \text{Height Factor} - \text{Age Factor}$$

Before we work out the answer, we must first calculate the Weight, Height, and Age Factors that go into the formula. These factors are computed differently for men and women.

To find your *Weight Factor*

1. Multiply your maintenance weight in pounds by 6.075
2. The answer is your Weight Factor

To find your *Height Factor*

1. Multiply your height in inches by 12.5
2. The answer is your Height Factor

To find your *Age Factor*

1. Multiply your age by 6.75
2. The answer is your Age Factor

Now that we have these three factors, we can go back to the formula and simply fill in the numbers. Here's how to do it:

1. Add 66.5 to your Weight Factor
2. Add your Height Factor to this answer
3. Subtract your Age Factor from that answer
4. Multiply that answer by .85
5. The resulting number is your daily metabolic rate
   (how many calories you burn without exercise)

FINDING YOUR TOTAL OUTPUT BY ADDING PHYSICAL ACTIVITY

Because you are moving around during the day and taking your Thermal Walks (see chapter 11), the total calories your body burns in a twenty-four-hour period is higher than your metabolic rate. To calculate your total output, we must add in this additional caloric burn-off.

To account for physical activity you must multiply your resting metabolic rate by 1.4. For example, if your resting metabolic rate is 1200 calories, you would multiply that number by 1.4 to obtain a total caloric output of 1680 calories per day.

This total output assumes that you are moderately active and are taking your Thermal Walks. If you are much less active and are not exercising, you would have to reduce this amount by at least 300 calories a day.

Depending on where you are on my Dietary Stairstepping ladder, you will have to recalculate your total caloric input each time you enter the Maintenance Stage at a different weight.

Now that you know how many calories you will burn during the Maintenance Stage, you also know how many calories you should eat. If you eat the same number of calories as you burn, you will not gain weight.

Having made all these calculations, I promise you that you'll never have to count calories again. You are now ready for the most important part of weight maintenance—my Portion Management System.

THE PORTION MANAGEMENT SYSTEM

Although there are several ways to manage calories while trying to maintain your weight, the easiest method is to keep a close eye on the size of your food servings. A major problem in dieting results from the fact that *most people underestimate the number of calories they eat.* In fact, people who follow a low-fat plan are especially prone to this problem because, without realizing it, they eat larger portions of low-fat foods.

Underestimating caloric intake is due primarily to the fact that *most people underestimate serving sizes by 50 percent or more!* A recent study at the University of Minnesota showed that errors in the estimation of portion sizes translated into miscalculations of several hundred calories and more than 10 fat grams a day. In another study, people who thought they were eating 2000 calories a day actually were eating 3000 calories. I have found that when people learn to identify appropriate serving sizes, they are much better able to control their weight.

MEASURING CUPS AND MENTAL IMAGERY

During the Weekday Low-Calorie and the Weekend Booster Stages, I asked you to measure all food portions. As you'll recall, this is one of the 6 Basic Rules of the New Hilton Head Metabolism Diet. This portion-size experience will now help you during the Maintenance Stage.

Portion Management requires measuring cups, measuring spoons, and a good food scale. As you measure and weigh foods each day you will quickly learn what a half a cup of cooked rice, three-quarters of a cup of cereal, or three ounces of chicken look like. You might even try to guess the size of a certain portion prior to measuring it and then see how accurate you are. This training at home will help you more accurately estimate portion sizes when you're eating out.

My clients at the Hilton Head Health Institute also find that using mental imagery to picture what various serving sizes look like is extremely helpful in judging portions. For example, you might visualize the following:

- 3 ounces of cooked meat is about the size of a deck of playing cards
- 1 1/2 ounces of hard cheese looks like three dominoes
- 1/2 cup of cooked pasta fits into an ice cream scoop
- 1/2 cup holds about 15 grapes
- 1 cup of cereal, chopped vegetables, or diced fruit is about the size of your closed fist
- 1 teaspoon of margarine or mayonnaise is about the size of the top joint of an average size person's thumb

As you measure foods, try to figure out other visual images that can help you with portion control.

HOW BIG A PORTION SHOULD YOU HAVE?

As a standard for comparison, the following is a list of everyday foods and the portion size that is considered 1 serving. These serving sizes are the approximate portions you would eat during your *weight loss* and will increase during weight maintenance.

1 Standard Serving

Bread.....................................1 slice or 1 small dinner roll

Cereal...................................1 ounce (1/2 to 1 cup depending on density of cereal)

Rice ....1/2 cup

Pasta.....................................1/2 to 1 cup, cooked (may be more with some recipes)

Potato...................................1/2

Vegetables (raw, leafy) ....1 cup

Vegetables (cooked or ....1/2 cup chopped)

Vegetable juice.......................6 ounces or 3/4 cup

Fruit (whole)..........................1 piece

Fruit (chopped).....................1/2 cup

Fruit juice..............................6 ounces or 3/4 cup

Milk ....8 ounces or 1 cup

Yogurt...................................1 cup

Cheese (hard).........................1 1/2 ounces

Lean meat...............................3 to 4 ounces

Fish ....4 to 6 ounces

Poultry ....3 to 4 ounces

As you probably noticed, the portions listed above are approximately those recommended in my menu plans for the Weekday Low-Calorie Stage and the Weekend Booster Stage.

During the Maintenance Stage you can easily increase calories in those menu plans by increasing portion sizes. The portion sizes that are appropriate for you will depend on your total caloric output, which we calculated earlier in this chapter. Now that you know your total output, simply look on the chart below for the portion sizes that are right for you.

PORTION MANAGEMENT CHART

Maintenance Calorie Level

Food Group	1500–1800	1800–2100	2100–2500
Bread (nondiet)	2 slices or 2 small rolls	2 slices or 2 small rolls	2 slices or 2 small rolls
Cereal	1 cup	1 1/4 cups	1 1/2 cups
Rice	3/4 cup	1 cup	1–1 1/2 cups
Pasta	3/4 to 1 cup	1 cup	1 1/2 cups
Vegetables (raw, leafy)	1 1/2 cups	2 cups	2–3 cups
Vegetables (cooked/ chopped)	1 cup	1 1/4 cups	1 1/2 cups
Potatoes	1/2 medium	1 whole medium	1 whole
Vegetable juice	8 ounces	10 ounces	12 ounces
Fruit (whole)	1 piece	1 1/2–2 pieces	2 pieces
Fruit (chopped)	3/4 cup	1 cup	1 1/2 cups
Fruit juice	8 ounces	10 ounces	12 ounces
Milk (1% or skim)	8 ounces	8 ounces	8 ounces
Low-fat yogurt	1 cup	1 cup	1 cup
Low-fat cheese	1 1/2 ounces	1 1/2 ounces	1 1/2 ounces
Low-fat cottage cheese	1/2 cup	1/2–3/4 cup	3/4–1 cup
Lean meat	4–5 ounces	6 ounces	7–8 ounces
Fish	4–6 ounces	6–8 ounces	7–9 ounces
Poultry	4–5 ounces	6 ounces	7–8 ounces
Salad dressing (low-fat)	2 tablespoons	2–3 tablespoons	2–3 tablespoons
Margarine (low fat)	1 teaspoon	1 teaspoon	1 teaspoon

USING THE PORTION MANAGEMENT CHART TO PLAN YOUR MAINTENANCE MENUS

To plan Maintenance Menus, all you have to do is adapt the Weekday Low-Calorie Menu Plan and the Weekend Booster Menu Plan by following these steps:

1. Increase serving sizes to correspond to the portion recommendations on the Portion Management Chart. Be sure you use the correct portion for your total caloric output. During the Maintenance Stage you will be eating the same number of calories on weekends as on weekdays. You will not need a Booster Weekend.

2. On days when there do not appear to be major differences between the low-calorie and maintenance portion sizes, increase calories by adding a roll or a salad to dinner or a glass of fruit or vegetable juice to a meal or minimeal.

3. Make sure you switch from low-calorie, diet bread to regular whole wheat bread, rolls, English muffins, or bagels during the Maintenance Stage. This will add calories without adding too much quantity.

4. If an increased portion size seems too large for you, you can increase calories by adding bread, fruit or vegetable juice, or a fruit and low-fat yogurt dessert. Or, eat half of the portion and include the other half in one of your later meals or minimeals.

5. When eating any food during the Maintenance Stage, at home or out, *do not exceed my portion size recommendations*. You may, however, eat a smaller portion than recommended. In addition, you may have noticed that my recommended pasta portions during the Low-Calorie and

Booster Stages are, at times, larger than the portion recommendations for the Maintenance Stage. This is because I am recommending the use of my low-calorie, low-fat recipes, which allow you larger portions than normally would be allowed when using regular recipes or when eating out. So, there are occasions when you will have to use your judgment and common sense. Eating a larger portion of fruit or vegetables from time to time is not a major problem. It would be, for foods that are higher in fat or calories.

6. When eating foods that contain *more than 2 to 3 grams of fat per 100 calories* (20 to 30 percent of calories from fat), limit your intake to very small portions. For example, if you choose to eat potato chips, you might limit yourself to one ounce, which is about two handfuls. Such foods should be consumed only occasionally.

If you follow my portion recommendations, you will be successful in maintaining your weight. Remember, during the Maintenance Stage:

- Measure all food eaten at home
- Use imagery to determine portion sizes when eating out
- Eat three meals and two minimeals every day and avoid eating at any other times
- Avoid high-fat foods, especially those containing more than 2 to 3 grams of fat per 100 calories
- If you occasionally choose to eat higher-calorie or higher-fat foods, keep portions to an absolute minimum.

Chapter 11
N N N

THE HILTON HEAD METABOLISM
EXERCISE PLAN

I f you're like most people, you realize that exercise is good for you. You also realize that exercise helps burn extra calories. Unfortunately, knowing these facts and doing something about them are two different things.

Many people, especially overweight people, dislike physical activity. Mere mention of the word *exercise* sends them into a panic. You may even be trying to figure out how to go on the New Hilton Head Metabolism Diet without exercising. Get those thoughts out of your head. I'm going to put you on the easiest exercise program of your life. I'm also going to show you how to get the *most* benefit out of the *least* amount of exercise.

If you don't particularly care for exercise, don't feel bad about it. It's not easy when you're carrying around thirty or forty extra pounds. You just can't move your body as easily as someone who is at his or her ideal weight. However, if you start out slowly and follow my plan, exercise will take on new meaning.

One of my clients had never in her life been physically active before she came to me. She avoided walking, drove her car even to visit a friend only one block away, and wouldn't have been caught dead in an exercise class. After four weeks on my program, she lost twenty pounds and was walking and bicycling every single day. Her husband and children couldn't believe it. She felt more energetic than she ever had and looked forward to her exercise. Now, two years later, she is keeping her weight off, walking every morning and riding an exercise bicycle every evening. She recently told me, "I can't believe the changes I've made. I can control my weight with just twenty minutes of exercise in the morning and twenty minutes in the evening. And the Metabolism Exercise Plan is easy. I don't have to strain. I go at my own pace and enjoy it. I actually look forward to my exercise. I feel like a new woman, inside and out."

Maybe it's not that you dislike exercise but that you're just not disciplined enough to stick to it. How many times have you vowed, "Today I'm going to start exercising. I'm fat, flabby, and out of shape. From now on I'm going to jog every day and work out at the health club three days a week"? So you start with an abundance of enthusiasm and the best of intentions. The first few days you push yourself to the limit. You forget that your muscles haven't been exercised in years. All of a sudden your body rebels. It's had it. You're sore all over. You can barely move. So you miss the next two days of exercise. And then it rains or the weather turns cold or you get too busy with the rest of your life. And that's the end of your exercise program.

Forget about the past. You've been going about this the wrong way. You've been trying to do too much too soon, perhaps even doing the wrong kinds of exercise. You may have been told that it takes so much exercise to burn fat that it's just not worth it. Besides, you're not a world-class marathoner and have no desire to become one.

Stop fretting and remember:

YOU DON'T HAVE TO SWEAT AND
STRAIN TO BURN FAT

That's right. You don't have to run to exhaustion or train for the Olympics to be slim and trim. Twenty minutes of moderate, "fun" exercise twice a day is all it takes.

WHY IS EXERCISE NECESSARY?

"Why can't I diet without exercising?" clients ask me. "I can lose weight without exercising. Besides, I've heard that it takes hours to burn off just one pound."

Well, if you want to increase your metabolism permanently, you must follow my exercise plan. You don't have to exercise for hours to get results. There are many misconceptions about physical activity and dieting. Forget everything you've ever heard and let me set you straight.

There are five reasons why exercise is *absolutely necessary* on the New Hilton Head Metabolism Diet.

1. Exercise Burns Calories

Whenever you are physically active, you burn additional calories. The best calorie-burning exercises are the simplest to do. Let's take walking as an example. Your jogging friends may tell you that walking is not strenuous enough to do you any good. That's nonsense! As far as calories are concerned, *walking is just as good as jogging*. In fact, walking burns as many calories as jogging. The number of calories your body burns during activity is related to the distance you travel, *not* how fast you go. This is so important for you to remember that I'm going to say it again:

The number of calories your body burns is related to the distance you travel, *not* how fast you go.

This is great news for dieters. You burn about 100 calories a mile whether you walk or run. The only difference is that the runner is finished faster. It would take a walker about twenty minutes to complete his mile, while a runner could do it in less than half that time. So what? What's ten minutes? Why not relax and enjoy burning your 100 calories in twenty minutes?

Many people are astonished by these facts. It's difficult to believe that runners do not burn a lot more calories per mile than walkers do. Now, don't confuse cardiovascular fitness with burning calories. More strenuous exercise, aerobic exercise, does condition the heart and lungs better than less strenuous exercise. But let's take one thing at a time. Your goal is to burn fat—to burn as much of it as you can. We'll worry about your fitness level later, *after* you lose your weight.

Another important element involved in burning calories through physical activity is your body size. This is one instance in which being bigger is better. As a general rule, the bigger you are, the more calories you burn during exercise. "Bigger" refers to your height *and* weight. A 160-pound person burns 104 calories while walking one mile. A 240-pound person burns 154 calories in the same distance. The reason is simple. Try carrying an 80-pound weight for one mile, and you'll discover how much extra effort and energy it takes.

2. Exercise Stimulates Your Metabolism

Exercise stimulates your metabolism and keeps it stimulated even after the exercise is over. These metabolic aftereffects can last several hours. So when you go for a mile walk, you're not just burning calories during that twenty-minute period. You're increasing the number of calories your body will burn for the next three or four hours. If you exercise twice daily, as I advise, you'll keep your metabolic furnace burning strong round the clock.

3. Exercise After Meals Doubly Stimulates Your Metabolism

Now I'm going to let you in on an essential bit of information that most doctors don't even know. For years my clients would ask me, "When is the best time of day to exercise?" My answer was that as long as you exercised regularly, it really didn't matter when you did it. Well, now I know that it *does* matter, and it matters a lot.

There is an important link between dietary thermogenesis and exercise. Thermogenesis, or the thermic effect, is the process by which your metabolism is stimulated after every meal you eat. Your metabolism burns calories at a faster rate for three to four hours after every meal. *Physical activity after meals doubles this thermic effect.* I can't stress to you enough how important this is.

By exercising *after* meals, you can increase the thermic stimulation of your metabolism from 25 percent to as much as 50 percent. Exercising after meals burns calories more efficiently than at any other time. You can't get as powerful an effect from your exercise or your meals in any other way. As you'll see, this mealtime-exercise connection is a basic underlying principle of my exercise plan.

4. Exercise Develops Muscle Tissue

Certain exercises, which I refer to as Muscle Firmers (see chapter 12), develop, tone, and firm muscle tissue. While they don't burn as much fat as the Thermal Walks (see p. 97), they are essential to metabolic efficiency. Your goal is to burn fat *and* develop muscle tissue.

Remember, the more muscle tissue, the higher your metabolism. You want to be as lean and as firm as you can get. If you just lose body fat without developing more muscle tissue, you won't change your metabolism nearly as much as you can and you won't look nearly as slim. I want you to burn every possible extra calorie. I want your body's furnace to be as finely tuned as possible.

I'm not saying you have to become a bodybuilder or that you have to be muscle-bound. You should be lean and firm. No more than 20 percent of your body weight should be fat if you are a man, and no more than 25 percent should be fat if you are a woman.

5. Exercise Gives You Energy

In addition to the physiological benefits of exercise on your metabolism, physical activity gives you a terrific energy boost. Regular exercise makes you feel alive and in control of your life. It helps you keep the commitment and motivation to follow my dietary plan.

Once you begin my exercise program, you'll soon feel a strong sense of confidence in yourself. You'll be back in control of your body again. All of your bodily processes, not just your metabolism, will function better with regular, moderate exercise.

THE HILTON HEAD METABOLISM EXERCISE PLAN

The Hilton Head Metabolism Exercise Plan is really quite simple and requires very little time. You will need to do two basic kinds of exercise: Thermal Walks and Muscle

Firmers. I will first describe Thermal Walks and give you the details of the Muscle Firmers in chapter 12.

THERMAL WALKS:
THE BEST WAY TO BURN CALORIES

A Thermal Walk is, by far, the most efficient way to burn fat and calories. This is also a very easy exercise for anyone to do regardless of weight. *A Thermal Walk is a 20-minute walk at a moderate pace that occurs after a meal.* As I said earlier, because of dietary thermogenesis:

AFTER-MEAL WALKING IS THE
MOST EFFICIENT WAY TO LOSE WEIGHT

Your daily weight management routine should consist of two Thermal Walks each and every day, without fail. To burn maximum calories you must schedule these after two of your five meals each day. It would be better to walk after one of your main meals rather than one of the minimeals. You will burn off more calories this way.

You should get into the habit of beginning your walk soon after your meal is finished. However, you can begin your walk up to an hour after the meal is finished and still get the effect. Keep in mind that the Thermal Walk should be a minimum of 20 minutes of continuous movement (no stopping along the way). It's perfectly okay if you want to walk for more than 20 minutes—just don't walk for any less.

You may walk outside or inside on a treadmill if you prefer. Walking is walking, so it really doesn't matter.

The pace of your walk is not important. Start at a moderate pace. Depending on your weight and fitness level, this could be a half-mile in 20 minutes, a mile, or, even faster. What's important here is that you walk for at least 20 minutes without stopping.

To summarize, here are your Thermal Walk guidelines:

1. Take two Thermal Walks after meals every day
2. Make sure each Thermal Walk lasts for at least 20 minutes
3. Don't wait longer than an hour after a meal to start your walk
4. Don't strain; moderation is the key
5. Try not to miss a day

Remember, Thermal Walks are not designed to be aerobic exercises. They are regular, moderate, consistent exercises that you perform day after day. Over your lifetime, you may have been told not to exercise after eating. Your mother may have required you to wait 30 minutes or so after eating to go for a swim. After-meal walking can cause problems only if you eat a very big meal and then walk very strenuously. In this case you are more likely to experience muscle cramping because the blood and oxygen needed by your muscles go instead to your gut to help digest the large meal you've just eaten. On this diet you will eat smaller meals, and the Thermal Walks should always be moderate. If you have any questions or concerns because of special medical problems, consult your physician.

Why Thermal Walks Are the Best Way to Lose Weight

Thermal Walks not only burn a lot of calories, but they are easy to stick to over a period of time. This was proven in a recent study at the University of Pittsburgh School of Medicine. In a study of 56 obese women, researchers found that the women who were allowed to break their exercise into shorter segments at various times in the day did better at sticking to their exercise plan than did the women who were required to do one 30- to 40-minute workout a day. After five months, the short-bout exercisers (similar to those on my two short Thermal Walk routine) had walked a total of 11 hours more than the once-a-day workout group and had also lost significantly more weight.

You do not have to exhaust yourself in one long workout three or four times a week in order to lose weight. You can succeed by following my twice-a-day moderate Thermal Walk routine, and the evidence suggests that you'll keep this pattern going week after week. If you choose to do a longer walk (for example, an hour) during the day I would still advise you also to do, at least, a 10 to 15 minute second walk.

Variations on the Thermal Walk

While I personally believe that walking is the best exercise of all, you may, from time to time, wish to vary your exercise routine. Perhaps, as a result of injury or illness, you may have to change the type of exercise you are doing. Acceptable alternatives to walking for your thermal activity may include bicycling (either outdoors or on an exercycle), swimming, dancing, or very low-level, low-impact aerobics. You could even walk around your home for 20 minutes doing chores. Just make sure not to keep starting and stopping.

COMMITMENT AND TIME

"All this talk about exercise is well and good, but I just don't have the time." This is the excuse I hear most frequently.

Believe me, I realize that you have to lead your normal life while dieting and exercising. I realize that it's not always easy.

I would suggest you consider your priorities in life. How important is it for you to lose weight and keep that weight off? If it is important, then you must schedule the time to do it right. *You* are important, and you're certainly worth it. You must make the time. It might take some re-arrangement of your schedule, but you *can* do it.

After all, I'm offering you a completely new way to lose weight. This is not just another diet but a way to improve your metabolism. This is the chance you've been waiting for. So don't hesitate. Make the time for yourself.

You'll find that once you get into the routine of Thermal Walks, my exercise plan will become second nature to you. Years ago, we had a cocker spaniel in the family named Albert. This dog was so much in the habit of our family Thermal Walks that whenever we cleared the dinner table after a meal, he would begin jumping up and down very excitedly looking forward to the walk.

PRECAUTIONS: EXERCISE AND YOUR HEALTH

Just one more note of caution. The exercise plan I've outlined is designed for people who are overweight but relatively healthy. If you have special medical problems such as heart trouble, high blood pressure, respiratory problems, or recurrent back pain, check with your physician before starting my exercise plan. He or she may want to advise you and periodically check your progress.

Thermal Walks should be done at a moderate pace. If you are breathing so hard that you cannot carry on a normal conversation, you're overdoing it.

Chapter 12

◪ ◪ ◪

MUSCLE FIRMERS

In addition to Thermal Walks, it will be necessary to add the Muscle Firmer exercises. Before you get upset about adding more exercises, let me assure you that I'm not adding any extra exercise time. You'll still be exercising twice a day for twenty minutes each session. That's the total amount of exercise time you'll ever need to keep you trim forever.

WHY ARE MUSCLE FIRMERS NECESSARY?

Your goal at the beginning of your diet is to burn as many calories as possible. This is best accomplished by using the Thermal Walks as I have instructed. To raise metabolism permanently, you must also develop as much muscle tissue as you can. While Thermal Walks develop some muscle tissue, their major function is to burn calories.

As you lose more weight, you must begin to add Muscle Firmers. These exercises don't burn as many calories, but they *do* firm, build, and tone muscle tissue. Remember, you want as much muscle tissue and as little body fat as possible. I'm not talking about being muscle-bound. I want your body to be lean and firm rather than fat and flabby. The basic idea behind the need for Muscle Firmers is:

THE MORE MUSCLE,
THE HIGHER YOUR METABOLISM

Muscle Firmers

The following are my 15 Muscle Firmers. You should schedule these exercises three times a week and, during busier times in your life, no less often than twice a week. You should always allow at least one day of rest between your scheduled exercise times. The Muscle Firmers should take about 20 minutes to complete. You should begin doing these exercises as well as the Thermal Walks as soon as you begin the diet.

Equipment You Will Need

In order to perform these exercises you will need a pair of hand-held weights or dumbbells. You will find a variety of these weights at your local discount or sporting-goods store. Any style will do. Some are the simple black iron variety while others are chrome. Many stores carry plastic-coated ones. Appearance doesn't matter, so the choice is up to you and your budget.

Choose a weight that is light enough for you to lift with one arm about 10 times without becoming overly fatigued. Women usually start out by using three- to five-pound weights, while men can often handle six to eight pounds. As you become stronger and firmer you will want to increase the size of the weights you are using. Just keep in mind that if you have to strain to complete these exercises, you are using too-heavy weight.

Number of Repetitions

You should strive to do 12 repetitions (one set) of each of the fifteen exercises. If you are not strong enough for 12 repetitions of any of the exercises, use a lighter weight. If you have the time and energy after completing one set, go through the fifteen exercises once again, doing 12 additional repetitions of each. Don't try to do more than the two sets of 12 repetitions.

Important Precautions

When performing Muscle Firmers, all movements should be slow and controlled, especially when lowering the weight. Don't be in a hurry, and don't use quick or jerky movements.

Make sure you breathe normally. It is very important that you do not hold your breath when doing these exercises.

The Correct Body Positions

For optimum safety and effectiveness, you must have your body positioned correctly when doing these exercises. Following are the three basic positions for the Muscle Firmers and which one to use for each exercise.

Straddle Stance Position

- Standing, start with your legs apart, slightly wider than shoulder width
- Center knees directly over heels (so you are not leaning forward, backward, or to one side)
- Point your toes slightly out to the side, bend your knees slightly, and contract the muscles in your stomach and buttocks

One Foot Forward Position

- Start in a comfortable standing position, then take a step back with one foot
- Center your knees over your heels
- Point your toes straight ahead, bend your knees slightly, and contract the muscles in your stomach and buttocks

On Your Back Position

- Lying on your back, start with your knees bent and your stomach muscles contracted
- Press your lower back downward so that it makes contact with the floor

THE 15 MUSCLE FIRMER EXERCISES

1. Bent Over Row

- Use the Straddle Stance position, with a weight in each hand
- Lean forward slightly from your hips, keeping your knees relaxed, your arms extended toward your feet, and your palms facing your body
- Pull the weights upward to the sides of your chest, keeping your elbows high
- Return to the starting position

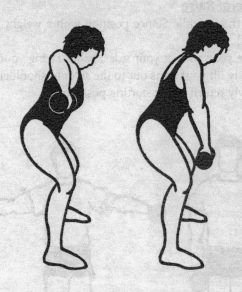

Bent Over Row

2. Lateral Raise

- Use the Straddle Stance position with a weight in each hand
- Place your arms at your sides, palms facing your body
- Slowly lift your arms out to the sides to shoulder height
- Slowly return to the starting position

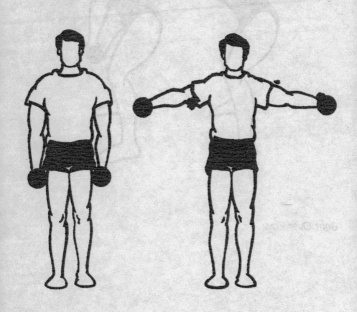

Lateral Raise

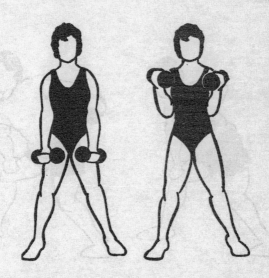

3. Upright Row

- Use the Straddle Stance position with a weight in each hand
- Place your arms down in front of your body with your palms facing your body
- Raise elbows out to the sides
- Slowly rotate your shoulders back
- Return to the starting position

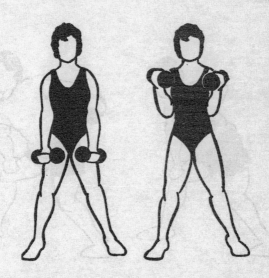

Upright Row

4. Kickbacks

- Use the One Foot Forward position, starting with your left foot forward and the weight in your right hand
- Place your left hand on your left thigh and lean forward slightly
- Extend your upper right arm back until your elbow is elevated and on an even level with your shoulder
- Extend arm to full length
- Return to the starting position and repeat on the other side

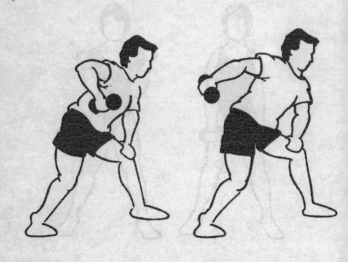

Kickbacks

5. Triceps Extension

- Use the One Foot Forward position, starting with your left foot forward and a weight in your right hand
- Slowly raise your right arm straight overhead from your shoulder
- Keep your elbow close to your head; bend your elbow and lower the weight behind your shoulder, supporting your right upper arm with your left hand
- Return to the starting position and repeat on the other side

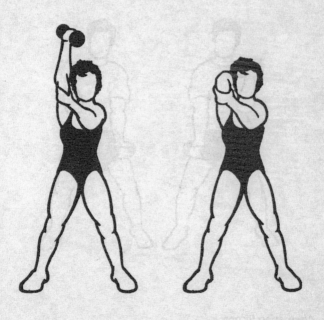

Triceps Extension

6. Alternating Biceps

- Use the Straddle Stance position with a weight in each hand
- With your elbows against your waist, extend your arms downward with your palms forward
- Lift your right hand toward your shoulder, then lower it to the starting position while you lift your left hand toward your shoulder
- Return to the starting position

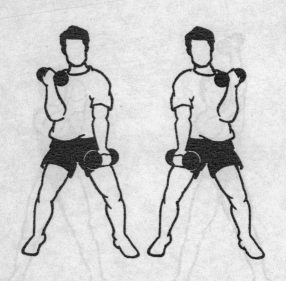

Alternating Biceps

7. Double Biceps

- Use the Straddle Stance position with a weight in each hand
- Holding your elbows against your waist, extend your arms downward with your palms forward
- Lift both hands toward your shoulders
- Return to the starting position

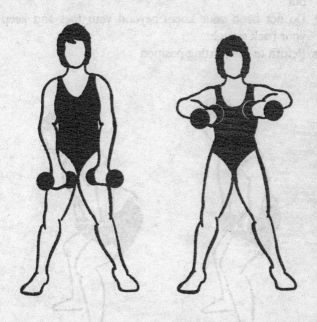

Double Biceps

8. Squats

- Use the Straddle Stance position with a weight in each hand
- Place your hands with the weights in them on your thighs
- Slowly bend your knees, shifting your weight back onto your heels, and allow your buttocks to push back and out
- Do not bend your knees beyond your toes and keep your back straight
- Return to the starting position

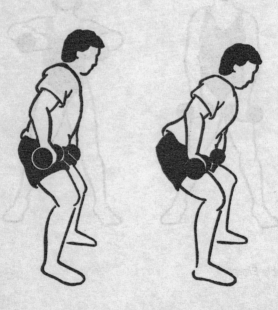

Squats

9. Heel Raises

- Use the Straddle Stance position but keep your toes forward rather than pointed to the sides
- With a weight in each hand extend your arms down to your sides
- Slowly rise up on your toes, lifting your heels off the floor
- Return slowly to the starting position

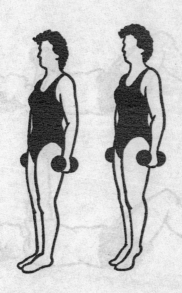

Heel Raises

10. Bench Press

- Use the On Your Back position with a weight in each hand
- Extend your arms on the floor to your sides
- Bend your elbows and raise your forearms even with your shoulders, with your palms forward
- Extend both arms straight up, then bend and return your elbows to the floor

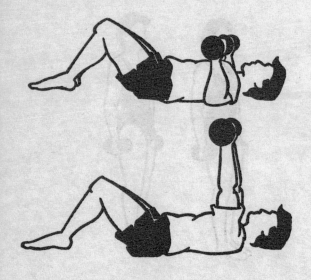

Bench Press

11. Chest Flys

- Use the On Your Back position with a weight in each hand
- Fully extend your arms, palms facing each other, and center the weights above your chest

  Slowly open your arms wide to your sides, keeping your elbows slightly bent (and your arms off the floor)

  Return to the starting position

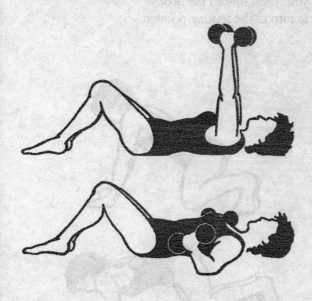

Chest Flys

12a. Box Push-ups

- (Use these push-ups if you are at a beginner's exercise level. No weights required.)
- Distribute your weight evenly on your hands and knees as shown in the illustration
- Center your hands under your shoulders with your knees under your hips
- Keeping your hips in place, bend at the elbows, moving your chest toward the floor
- Return to the starting position

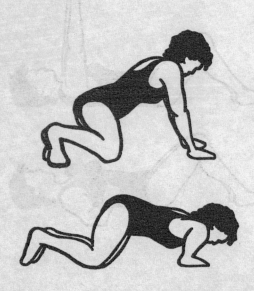

Box Push-ups

12b. Extended Push-ups

(Use these push-ups if you are stronger or a more experienced exerciser. No weights required.)

- Extend your body so that your weight is distributed between your hands and your toes
- Keeping your body and head aligned, lower your body to the floor
- Return to the starting position

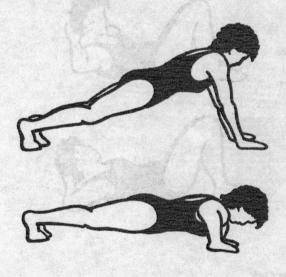

Extended Push-ups

13. Upper Curls (no weights required)

- Use the On Your Back position
- Place your hands behind your head, keeping your elbows wide
- Raise your head and shoulders off the floor
- Return halfway to the floor

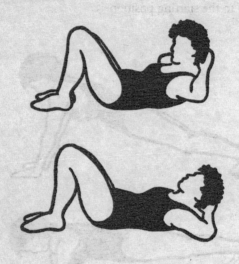

Upper Curls

14. Oblique Curls (no weights required)

- Use the On Your Back position
- Hold your arms at your sides, raised a few inches off the floor
- Hold your head and shoulders slightly off the floor
- Extend your right hand toward the toes of your right foot
- Return to the original position and extend your left hand toward the toes of your left foot

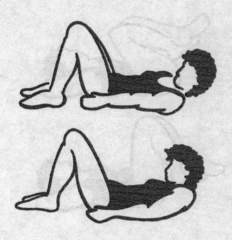

Oblique Curls

15. Reverse Curls (no weights required)

- Use the On Your Back position
- Place your hands behind your head
- Keep your head and shoulders flat on the floor
- Lift your hips back toward your head until your bent knees move slowly toward your chest and your feet come off the floor
- Slowly release back down

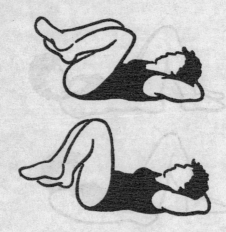

Reverse Curls

MUSCLE FIRMERS ARE A MUST

Because building muscle tissue is so important for your metabolism, doing these resistance exercises two to three times a week is essential. Remember, the amount of muscle in your body is highly correlated with metabolic rate, so by increasing muscle tissue you are adding extra metabolic horsepower. Muscle Firmers also make you stronger and give your body a firmer, younger appearance. It is essential that you do both the Thermal Walks *and* the Muscle Firmers in order to stimulate your metabolism to the fullest.

Chapter 13

N N N

QUESTIONS AND ANSWERS ABOUT THE HILTON HEAD METABOLISM EXERCISE PLAN

These are the most commonly asked questions about my exercise plan:

Q. *I live in a very cold climate. How can I walk when it's so cold and snowy?*

A. Walking in very cold weather actually speeds up your metabolism even more and burns more calories. If it's simply too cold, snowy, or rainy to walk outside, try dancing to music, exercycling, or indoor rowing.

Q. *Why haven't you mentioned jumping rope or jogging in place?*

A. While these exercises are good for developing cardiovascular fitness, they are potentially harmful to anyone who is overweight. The repeated jolting of your body against the floor puts undue strain on your legs, knees, ankles, and feet. If you have any kind of back trouble, you should be particularly careful of these exercises.

Q. *I am fifty-five years old, forty pounds overweight, and haven't exercised in years. Are there any precautions I should take before going on your exercise plan?*

A. Yes. You definitely should consult your physician before starting any exercise program, especially at your age and weight. He or she may want to administer a treadmill electrocardiogram test (often called a stress test) to check out your heart. Your doctor also may want you to start out very slowly, perhaps walking only a quarter or a half mile until you become more accustomed to exercise.

Q. *I attend an aerobic dancing class three days a week. Could I eat my lunch thirty minutes before class on these days and count this as one of my metabolism exercise sessions?*

A. Definitely, yes. This would be a fine idea. The more you can incorporate my plan into your regular routine, the better.

Q. *Is it all right to do the same type of exercise twice a day? I find it easier to hop on my indoor exercise bike after meals every day.*

A. It's perfectly okay to use the same exercise each day. Some people are more consistent if they keep up exactly the same exercise routine. Other people need more variety in their lives and like to vary the exercises. Either way will do.

Q. *Would you suggest that I do your exercises alone or together with someone else?*

A. Again, it depends on your personality. If you are a "people" person, then by all means find an exercise partner. Couples who are dieting together often enjoy exercising together. They enjoy having someone to talk to. On the other hand, some people use their exercise times to relax and "get away from it all." They prefer to be alone during exercise, so that they can unwind, meditate, or let their minds wander.

Q. *I lead a very active life. I'm on the go all the time, with car pools for the children, shopping, and running errands. Why do I need to exercise after all this activity?*

A. I'm sorry to say that your "running around" all day counts very little as a calorie-burning activity. For physical activity to burn fat, it must be continuous and timed right (e.g., *after* meals). Your stop-and-go car pools and shopping are not enough.

Q. *I'm so worn out after my workday that I don't have enough energy for your exercise plan. How can I exercise when I'm exhausted?*

A. Probably the most frequent complaint I hear from my overweight clients is that they lack energy. My diet and exercise program will give you more energy than you've had in years. After a busy day, exercise will give you *more* energy, even though you may feel exhausted. If you exercise for twenty minutes after dinner, I promise that you won't fall asleep on the couch watching television as you usually do. You'll feel rejuvenated. Remember that much of the fatigue you feel after work may be mental rather than physical.

Q. *Although I am about twenty pounds overweight, I jog three miles every day at an eight-minute-per-mile pace. Do I have to schedule my run after a meal?*

A. I do not recommend strenuous exercising after meals unless it occurs thirty minutes after a very light meal such as the minimeal. Schedule your jogging for anytime you like. However, I would still suggest my Thermal Walks after two of your four meals. These should be moderately paced and not strenuous.

Q. *When you say I should exercise twenty minutes after a meal, is that the length of time after the beginning or end of my meal?*

A. You should estimate the time based on the end of your meal.

Q. *What if I feel like exercising for more than twenty minutes after a meal?*

A. If you have the time and the inclination, by all means, walk or bike a little farther. Just don't overdo it.

Q. *What if I'm eating dinner out and can't start my exercise until one or two hours after the meal?*

A. If two hours have elapsed, I would suggest that you exercise after your next meal. However, if it's your last meal of the day and you've had only one other exercise time, then you should exercise, regardless of the time.

Q. *Will your exercise get rid of cellulite in my thighs and hips?*

A. Probably the biggest hoax perpetrated on the American public is the concept of cellulite. Cellulite is supposed to be a special, dimply kind of fat that women get on their hips and thighs. The truth of the matter is that cellulite is simply normal, everyday fat. It's the same kind of fat that you have in the rest of your body. Some people inherit a tendency to have more fat in the lower portion of their bodies. The lumpy, dimpling effect is simply caused by the size and spacing of fat cells. Such fat can be removed only by dieting. Exercise will firm muscles in the thighs and hips, and dieting will burn the fat.

Chapter 14

◙ ◙ ◙

IMPROVING YOUR WILLPOWER: HOW TO OVERCOME FOOD CRAVINGS AND OUT-OF-CONTROL EATING

Out-of-control eating, or bingeing, can be a significant problem when trying to control your weight. While most people think of binge eating as being exclusive to eating disorders, 50 percent of those who are overweight binge occasionally, with about 25 percent bingeing frequently.

What exactly is binge eating? It is defined as the intake of a large amount of food in a short period of time, characterized by a feeling of *loss of control*. If you show this pattern of behavior, it is important to identify and overcome it, since out-of-control eating is a serious obstacle to successful weight control.

WILLPOWER OVER FOOD CAN BE LEARNED

Anyone can develop more willpower over food by using my Willpower Training system. Willpower is not something that you are born with or without. It is a skill that is learned, although most people haven't the faintest idea how to go about learning it.

I want you to realize that willpower is simply the ability to resist eating tempting foods or to resist eating when you are under emotional stress. I'm not just talking about "toughing it out." Willpower Training conditions you both biochemically and emotionally so that you are no longer as tempted by fatty or sweet foods.

The specific goals of Willpower Training are:

1. To teach you to distinguish between real hunger and food cravings based on emotions
2. To desensitize you to the sights and thoughts of tempting foods so that your body loses its craving reaction

WILLPOWER TRAINING, PART 1: BREAKING THE LINK BETWEEN HUNGER AND EMOTIONS

Many dieters have difficulty differentiating between hunger and emotions. You might wrongly interpret feelings such as fatigue, boredom, restlessness, and tension as hunger rather than as the emotions they really are. For you, boredom and hunger may have the same meaning. Whenever you are emotionally upset, you may assume that your body is telling you that it's time to eat.

You can break the connection between hunger and emotions by:

1. Learning to pay more attention to what *real* hunger is and what it feels like
2. Not allowing yourself to use food as a psychological drug to calm tension or relieve hurt feelings

By establishing a routine schedule for meals, you will gradually teach yourself to be hungry when it is appropriate to be hungry—that is, after a period of time has gone by without eating. If, after a few days on the New Hilton Head Metabolism Diet, you feel hungry twenty minutes prior to a meal, you should be pleased. By eating only at certain times, your body has been conditioned to feel real hunger. This is great news and provides an excellent opportunity to analyze your hunger sensations.

I want you to realize that there is nothing wrong with feeling hungry. It is not a *bad* feeling, just a natural one that is slightly unpleasant but only temporarily so. In fact, you could begin to think of hunger as a *good* experience. It shows that you are sticking to your eating plan, and it gives you the chance to examine hunger and learn more about it. Once you learn what hunger really feels like, you can learn to control it without fearing it.

When you are experiencing hunger, use the opportunity to ask yourself these questions:

- What does my stomach feel like? Does it feel empty? Is it growling? Is it contracting?
- What does my mouth feel like? Is my mouth watering? Are my jaws tense or tight?
- What other physical sensations do I have?

Try to focus on physical rather than emotional feelings.

Once you set your schedule of meals and minimeals for a particular day, do not change it because of your hunger. If you're hungry between meals and believe your hunger is emotionally based, use that opportunity to focus on what you are feeling. Get out a piece of paper or a notebook and write down what you are experiencing. What emotion is it? Are you angry, sad, tense, depressed, bored? Write down your emotional reactions or talk them out with someone. Keep in mind that food is a nutrient for your body, not a drug to alleviate bad feelings.

Search for other ways to deal with these feelings. Instead of eating, you might go for a walk, talk to a friend or loved one, take a few deep breaths, get out of the house for a while, or distract yourself with a favorite activity. Just don't eat, whatever you do. Actually, one of the best stress-management tools is exercise. You'll be getting rid of stressful emotions and excess calories at the same time.

WILLPOWER TRAINING, PART 2: DESENSITIZING YOURSELF TO THE SIGHT OF HIGH-CALORIE FOODS

Willpower Training is designed to break the conditioned biochemical processes that occur when you are tempted by your favorite foods. The power of food cravings can be enormous. Dr. Judith Rodin of Yale University studied overweight and nonoverweight people while they were being tempted by their favorite foods. She found that people who are overweight, whether or not they have just eaten, experience strong bodily reactions to the mere sight of appetizing food. For example, she discovered that when you look at tempting food and think about it, your pancreas begins to secrete insulin. One effect of increased insulin output is a decrease in blood sugar level, which in turn is associated with feelings of hunger, especially cravings for sweets.

In other words, the *psychological* temptation triggers a bodily reaction that brings about a real *physiological* hunger for food. This reaction is more prevalent in those who are overweight, especially those who have been overweight since childhood. Because of this strong connection between the sight of food and physical reactions, you must begin the process of deconditioning by building your willpower.

The basic notion behind Willpower Training is that the more you avoid favorite foods or the more they are withheld from you, the more tempting they become. The "forbidden fruit" is the most tempting of all. Besides, in our society, there is absolutely no way to avoid tempting foods, as we are exposed to them every day.

Willpower Training for control over eating is a bit like training someone to overcome a phobia. Since a phobia is an unrealistic fear, such as the fear of heights or elevators or bugs, the way to get over it is gradually to accustom yourself to the feared situation, little by little. In this way you desensitize yourself to the object of your anxiety, gain self-confidence, and lose your fear.

The same is true with cravings for food. By confronting your temptations, first in imagination and then in real life, you can gradually gain control over your reactions. Over time, your body will stop responding so strongly to the sight of these temptations. It's a bit like learning any other skill: you practice willpower little by little until you become an expert at it.

During Willpower Training you will be using your imagination to think about situations in which you are being tempted to eat. This imaginary exposure to food should last five to ten minutes, every day for at least two weeks, and then as often as you think you need it.

Close your eyes and think of a food that is very appealing. Make certain that it is a high-calorie food. It could be any type of food—ice cream, candy, doughnuts, fried

chicken, cheese, potato chips, or any other of your favorites. Now imagine that you are being tempted by that
food. Visualize the scene in great detail. For example, you
might be in the kitchen by yourself looking into a con-
tainer of chocolate ice cream. Use all of your senses (except
taste). Try to see all aspects of the food. Look at it. Smell it.
Let your imagination go as you pretend you are really in
that particular situation.

However, it is very important that during these training sessions you:

NEVER IMAGINE YOURSELF
EATING THE TEMPTING FOOD

Remember, you are practicing how to resist food, not how
to eat it.

During these sessions, go through one or two scenes
several times. You will find that each time you imagine the
tempting situation, it will be easier to overcome the imaginary food craving.

After one or two days of practice, make it more difficult by practicing when you are actually hungry or are
emotionally upset. Use as many tempting-food situations
as you can think of, trying to duplicate as many real-life
occurrences as possible.

The following is an example of an imaginary food
scene.

On the kitchen table, right in front of you, is a bag of
the cheese-flavored snacks that you love so much. You are
so hungry. You realize that in an hour you are going to have
a planned, low-fat meal, but right now you'd love to have

the cheese snacks. The longer you look at them, the more you want them. You can feel the hunger building in your body. Concentrate on how much you want the food and how your craving is making you feel.

Although you really want the snacks, *you do not eat them*. Take a slow, deep breath. Breathe in slowly through your nose and slowly let it out through your mouth. Relax. Try to feel yourself relax and imagine the craving slowly going away. You are feeling strong, with a great deal of willpower.

You walk out of the kitchen, leaving the snacks where they are. You go into another room, feeling relaxed and calm. You feel good about yourself, with a strong sense of success and accomplishment. You proved to yourself that you had willpower, that you were stronger than the food. You take another slow, deep breath and relax even more.

Each visualization exercise helps to further desensitize your food temptations. Even though these are imaginary successes, the experiences build confidence and enable you to overcome real food cravings.

Use these willpower visualizations before going into a tempting-food situation. If you're going to a party where there will be lots of food and drink, imagine yourself there, being tempted by the food, but not giving in. Then, imagine how strong and positive you'll feel after the party, having chosen the healthful foods and avoiding the fatty or sweet ones.

If you slip up from time to time and succumb to temptation, practice imaginary food exposure after the fact. Imagine yourself being tempted once again, but this time you avoid the food or eat only a small portion.

If you practice Willpower Training diligently, you'll be amazed at the results. I've had people tell me that this training has completely changed their attitude toward food and given them a new sense of power and control over food cravings. The secret lies in practice and lots of it.

Chapter 15

◪ ◪ ◪

KEEPING YOUR MOTIVATION HIGH

Keeping yourself motivated is an important key to losing weight. Since the New Hilton Head Metabolism Diet is based on such a revolutionary concept, motivation is usually not a problem. Once you understand my approach and get started on the diet, you will feel a sense of enthusiasm and motivation that will carry you through to your goal. And remember, your goal is not simply to lose weight. Your goal is to change your metabolism permanently so that you will be able to eat normally, maybe for the first time in your life. The knowledge that you really are able to change your body chemistry forever will keep you on the program day after day.

Being human, you may experience brief lapses in motivation from time to time. This is especially true if you have a lot of weight to lose. Here are some hints on how to keep your motivation high.

KEEPING YOUR GOALS IN MIND

The number one thing you must guard against is *impatience*. You will want your excess weight to disappear in a few days. Just like many of life's other challenges, dieting requires time and patience. You must give it a chance to work.

By keeping your eventual weight goal in mind, you can ward off these feelings. Start by figuring out the specific reasons you are trying to lose weight and to lose it forever. Consider both the short-term and long-term future. What are the advantages to *you*, personally, to lose weight?

To help you answer this question, let's imagine that you have already lost your weight. You are slim and trim and have been that way for one full year. You feel totally in control of your weight. You are able to eat normally without gaining weight. As you think this pleasant thought, make a list of as many advantages of being slim and trim as you can think of. Try to make them personally relevant.

Write your list on an index card, so you can keep it handy. One of my patients came up with the following list of pluses.

- I would feel more attractive.
- I would feel proud of myself and have more self-confidence.
- I would be less moody and not as likely to feel resentful, sensitive, angry, and depressed.
- I would be able to wear smaller-size and more stylish clothes.
- I would feel more outgoing and be more socially active.
- I would have a more enjoyable sex life and not be ashamed of my body.
- I would be more physically active and more involved in recreational activities.
- I would live longer and lessen the likelihood of being disabled by a stroke or heart attack.
- I would serve as a good example to others, particularly my children.

Keep this list in a prominent place at home. Put it where you will see it every day. Every few days during the diet, and especially when your motivation is low, read the list over very carefully. Read each item and think about it. Then pick one or two for more intense consideration.

Let's suppose you pick the one about clothes fitting better. Now close your eyes and imagine that you have already lost your weight. Visualize yourself walking into one of your favorite clothing stores. As you look at the clothes in your "new," smaller size, select an outfit that you find attractive. Make sure it is one that will show off your figure. How about a swimsuit? Now go into the dressing room and try the outfit on. Come out and look at yourself in the mirror. The outfit really flatters your new shape. You look terrific! Try to imagine what you would actually be feeling. What a sense of accomplishment! Look at your lean body. Feel the exhilaration and pride. Let yourself experience the excitement of the moment.

It's important to visualize this scene as clearly and as vividly as you can. Use all of your senses. See, hear, feel, and touch what is happening. Use a different item on your list each time you practice visualization. After your little mental trip into the future, you will feel a renewed, strong sense of commitment and a much greater resolve.

EXCUSES, EXCUSES, EXCUSES

From time to time we all use the darnedest excuses to avoid exercise or to eat more calories than we should. It is human nature to give yourself an "acceptable" reason for not sticking to your plan of action. What is even more frustrating is the fact that we all use the *very same* excuses over and over again. It is only later, after you have overeaten or missed your exercise, that you see through the flimsy excuse.

You must be aware of your excuses, identify them for what they are, and counterattack with a stronger argument.

Here are some typical excuses along with a counterattack for each. If you hear yourself making an excuse, immediately replace it with a more positive counterattack thought.

Excuse 1. But I have tried other diets and failed. It is just impossible for me to lose weight.

Counterattack. The reason I failed before is because I went about it the wrong way. The New Hilton Head Metabolism Diet is completely different. This is finally my chance to succeed.

Excuse 2. I have been just as faithful to the diet as my husband has, and he is losing faster than I am. I am getting discouraged.

Counterattack. Men are supposed to lose faster than women because of their higher metabolic rates. Besides, the reason I am on this program is because my metabolism is sluggish. If I give it a chance, my metabolism will pick up, and I will be burning more calories than I ever have before.

Excuse 3. It is impossible to schedule all these meal and exercise times with a schedule like mine.

Counterattack. Nothing is impossible if I want it badly enough. I may have to do some creative time management, but *I can do it.*

Excuse 4. I don't have any willpower.

Counterattack. I don't need any more willpower than anyone else. Willpower is simply planning ahead and wanting to succeed. Besides, the New Hilton Head Metabolism Diet is easy to follow, and I don't have to be a saint to stick to the rules.

Excuse 5. I am too nervous and upset right now. I will just have to get off the diet and get back on it later.

Counterattack. Being nervous and upset about things happening in my life should have nothing to do with dieting and exercise. Good nutrition and regular exercise help me cope with the stresses, strains, and emotional upsets of life. Being depressed or upset or angry is *not* a good reason to eat or skip exercise. What I should be doing is trying to solve the problem, finding a sympathetic friend who will lend an ear, or learning better skills to deal with emotional stress.

Excuse 6. I hate dieting. I always feel so deprived.

Counterattack. The New Hilton Head Metabolism Diet is different. I really do not feel deprived. It is a positive approach. I feel that for the first time in my life I am doing the right thing to control my weight. I feel positive and satisfied with the diet.

Excuse 7. I am going on vacation for a week. I will just have to get back on the diet when I come home.

Counterattack. I *can* vacation and diet at the same time. The New Hilton Head Metabolism Diet fits easily into any schedule. In fact, it may be even easier on vacation because my time is my own.

Excuse 8. Everybody else at this party is eating and drinking whatever they want. It's not fair that I have to diet.

Counterattack. My diet is only temporary. And the faster I get my metabolism back to normal, the faster I will be able to eat like everyone else. If I give in now, it will only slow my progress and take my metabolism longer to get into shape.

FRIENDLY ENEMIES

Your family and friends can have a tremendous effect on your motivation. They can encourage you and help you keep going. On the other hand, they can do or say things that have the reverse effect. If you have ever gone off a diet out of anger or spite, then you know exactly what I am talking about. There are four particularly damaging types of remarks you sometimes hear from family and friends.

Critical Remarks

Critical remarks about you or your diet can be quite discouraging. Ever hear such comments as, "Oh no, not another diet!" or (especially on the New Hilton Head Metabolism Diet), "Spaghetti!? I never heard of a diet that allows that. Are you sure you're not cheating?"

Pessimistic Remarks

Some people react negatively to just about everything, but especially to diets. They will try to discourage you by saying, "No diet is permanent. You will just gain it all back," or, "I know you will never last more than a few days."

Permissive Remarks

Some people feel sorry for you. In an attempt to be "nice" they give you excuses to go off the diet (as if you didn't have enough of your own). They say, "Go ahead. That ice cream won't hurt you," or, "Don't worry. It doesn't matter if you don't exercise for a couple of days." Sometimes these are overweight friends looking for company.

Supervisory Remarks

Probably the most infamous of all friendly enemies is what I call the *dietary supervisor*. This person tries to "help" you by taking control of your diet. He or she assumes that since you have failed at diets before, you need someone to look after you. They advise you, push you, and remind you. They say, "Don't forget to do your exercise today," or, "Now let's make sure *this* diet works," or, "Now don't be eating anything you're not supposed to today." These remarks only make you want to eat more, exercise less, and throw something (preferably something large and heavy) at your self-appointed supervisor.

The difficult part about dealing with these comments is that they usually come from those who care about you the most. Keep in mind that these people are trying to help you. They are not hostile, vindictive, or out to get you. They are just misguided. They simply do not understand dieting, and they may not understand you very well either. Just don't be overly sensitive to their comments. Remind yourself that their intentions are good, but that they just don't understand.

When these remarks occur often or when these comments make it more difficult for you to stick to the diet, you may have to let people know how they are affecting you. Don't be shy. Just tell them in a direct, straightforward manner that, even though they are trying to help, their remarks are having a negative effect. You must convince them that for you to succeed, *you* and you alone must be responsible for that success. You want their encouragement, of course, but not their criticism, advice, or supervision.

Also, ask family members *not* to:

- Tease you about your diet
- Offer you foods you are not supposed to eat
- Repeatedly ask how many pounds you have lost
- Give you advice
- Remind you to stick to your diet
- Admonish or lecture you if you "slip"

TEMPORARY SETBACKS

What should you do if in spite of your best efforts you slip up a bit? First, remember that you are human and subject to error from time to time. A slip does *not* mean you are a failure. It does *not* mean you don't have willpower. It simply means you are human, like everyone else. Second, do *not*, under any circumstances, allow yourself to feel guilty. Guilt will just make you feel worse and keep you from getting back on the straight and narrow.

Avoid such thoughts as, "Well, I have really blown it now. Maybe I'll get back on the program next week." Get back on the program *immediately*. In fact, try not to think in terms of being *on* or *off* the diet. If you slip, consider it a slight deviation from the plan. You are only slightly off course. Do not act as if your ship has sunk.

Profit from your mistakes. If you missed your after-meal exercise today, figure out what went wrong. How could you have gotten your exercise in? Could you have arranged your schedule differently? Once you have figured this out, forget about your slip. Turn your mistake into a good lesson.

Never, ever compensate for a slip by missing a meal. Even if you eat a candy bar at 4:00 P.M., eat your dinner as planned. Remember, skipping meals is a very, very bad habit and especially bad for your metabolism. If you feel a need to undo your wrongdoing, exercise a little more that day or the next.

I believe you will find the New Hilton Head Metabolism Diet so different and so challenging that slips will rarely occur. You will feel positive, and you will make progress every day. You *can* do it. I want to make this the last diet of your life. I have faith in you. Just remember to have faith in yourself.

Chapter 16
✖ ✖ ✖
BEING REALISTIC ABOUT DIETING

You don't have to become a hermit to stick to the New Hilton Head Metabolism Diet. I want you to live your life exactly the way you do when you're not dieting. That means at restaurants and dinner parties and on business trips and vacations. If you avoid these situations, you'll feel "different" and deprived. You'll soon become bored and restless and feel sorry for yourself. And before you know it, there goes the diet. So, you must get used to dealing with every possible eating situation.

WATCH YOUR ATTITUDE

Forget about your past diets and past failures. Since the New Hilton Head Metabolism Diet emphasizes calories burned up more than calories eaten, you can stay on the diet and live a normal life at the same time. You don't have to panic about eating out.

On other diets you may have had a tendency to get lax when not eating at home. Perhaps it was easy to give yourself an excuse for going off the diet. You may have thought, "How can anyone diet at a dinner party? It's unheard of!"

I'm telling you it's not only possible, it's easy. Remember:

NO EATING SITUATION EXISTS
THAT YOU CANNOT HANDLE

Don't be afraid or give up when you eat out. View the experience as a *challenge*. Accept the challenge and face it head on. The New Hilton Head Metabolism Diet menus can easily be adapted to *any* situation.

RESTAURANTS

The first rule in dealing successfully with restaurants is to plan ahead. Try to choose a restaurant with a varied menu. Ethnic restaurants are fine occasionally, but they make it much more difficult for you to stick to the diet.

It also helps to plan out the exact type of meal you will order. This is a lot easier if you are familiar with the restaurant you're going to. The first step in this planning process is to look at my menus to determine what you're supposed to have that day. If possible, plan to order exactly what I have prescribed. Slight variations of vegetables or fruits are certainly allowed.

If you feel you'll have difficulty ordering the meal for that day, simply choose the corresponding meal from another day.

Here are some basic restaurant rules for you to keep in mind.

- Always make sure to order your fish broiled *without* butter.
- Don't be hesitant to ask about portion sizes—e.g., how many ounces is the chicken or fish? If the serving is more than the diet calls for, put the extra to the side of your plate.

- If you order meat, make sure you cut off all visible fat before eating it.
- If your menu calls for diet margarine on the potato but the restaurant doesn't carry it, use half the amount of regular margarine.
- Make sure that no sauces are added to your entree. You may have to give the waiter or waitress specific instructions about this.
- Make sure no salad dressing, croutons, or bacon bits are added to your salad.
- Order your vegetables plain, with no butter or sauce added.
- If you order chicken, remove the skin before eating it.
- Order fresh fruit for dessert if it's available. If they have only canned fruit, forget it. Canned fruit is usually packaged in sugary syrup. If they don't have fruit and your menu calls for it, have extra fruit at home with your minimeal.
- Since salt is used freely in restaurant kitchens, do not add salt when you're eating out. You may retain extra fluid, which will temporarily add weight.
- Ask questions of the waiter or waitress and be specific about exactly what you want.
- You are the customer; you are paying the bill; it's their job to accommodate you.

If you end up at a specialty or ethnic restaurant, you can still order something that is low in fat and calories. You may have difficulty sticking strictly to the menus I have outlined; try to abide by them with as few variations as possible.

Italian restaurants are adaptable to the diet, since they serve veal, chicken, and pasta dishes, all of which are acceptable on the diet. It's the cheeses, stuffings, sauces, and wine you must avoid. Veal Piccata (with lemon and wine sauce) is an excellent entree and is only 300 calories (about 4 ounces).

While my wife, Gabrielle, was in the process of losing thirty pounds some time ago (pounds she has never gained back), we ate in a popular Italian restaurant in New York City. She first ordered a small salad with vinegar as the dressing. For her entree she ordered a stuffed lamb chop. She ate the chop and left the stuffing. The lamb chop was accompanied by green beans, which she ordered without butter. The waiter was at first a bit taken aback by her apparent lack of appetite for the special "dishes of the house," but, after a little explanation and joking back and forth, he was extremely accommodating. He could have lost a few pounds himself, and by the end of our dinner he seemed quite in awe of her willpower.

Another excellent choice in Italian restaurants is spaghetti. Just make sure the tomato sauce contains no meat and that you ask for a small portion. Remember, you can even have the Italian bread with your spaghetti dinner. Doesn't sound like being deprived, does it?

Chinese food can be okay if you're careful. If you have high blood pressure or retain fluid easily, watch out for the soy sauce and the monosodium glutamate (MSG). Generally speaking, Chinese food is low in calories. However, avoid egg rolls, dumplings, and spareribs. Stick to dishes that are boiled, steamed, or poached rather than stir-fried with oil. Avoid pork and sausage dishes. Chicken or shrimp dishes are probably your best bets. I would suggest Chicken subgum (chicken with vegetables), Egg foo yong, or chicken with snow peas. Avoid any dishes with nuts.

French restaurants are a particular challenge because of their penchant for sauces loaded with cream, butter, and eggs. Avoid these sauces while dieting, because the fat and calories are deadly. A simply prepared grilled fish such as a striped bass is a good choice. Roast chicken (*Poularde Rotie*), medallions of beef (*Medallions de Filet de Boeuf*), or peppered filet mignon (*Filet Mignon au Poivre Flambé*) are excellent meals for your diet. The entree can be accompanied by a vegetable (no sauce, please) and a potato (baked, not French fried). For dessert you can have fresh fruit (plain, with no topping), which is readily available in most French restaurants.

DINNER PARTIES

You must also be able to contend with dinners at the homes of friends or business associates. In these situations your choices are more limited than in restaurants, but don't worry, you can handle it. Small dinners with intimate friends are often easier, since most friends will know you're dieting and try to accommodate you. Maybe you'll be really lucky, and your friends will join you on the New Hilton Head Metabolism Diet. One of my clients arrived at a friend's dinner party and, to her delight and relief, was served a dinner from the Booster Weekend Menu, exactly as I described it. It seemed that the hostess had just begun the New Hilton Head Metabolism Diet two weeks earlier and was determined to stick to my plan in spite of her dinner party. Everyone enjoyed the meal and no one, except my client, knew they had just enjoyed a diet meal.

Don't panic if the dinner party starts out with cocktails and hors d'oeuvres. Arrive a little late and quickly get yourself a club soda with lime or lemon. Position yourself as far away from the hors d'oeuvres as possible, and get involved in an interesting conversation. As you watch others eating and drinking, try to feel a little superior to them. You are changing your metabolism while they continue to suppress theirs. Go ahead. It's okay to feel snobbish. After all, you've found the secret to dieting success once and for all.

If the dinner party is like most I've attended, be prepared to eat later than usual. To prepare for this, I suggest you have your minimeal in the late afternoon, even if you typically have it later, after dinner. You might also plan to eat lunch later that day, say around 1:30 P.M., then not have your minimeal until 5:30 P.M. Also, make sure you get your after-meal exercises in early that day. You may not eat dinner until 9:00 or 9:30 P.M., and you'll probably sit around socializing afterward. By the time you arrive home, it's doubtful you'll exercise. So plan your Thermal Walks or other energy-burning exercises after breakfast and lunch.

If the dinner is served buffet style, you'll at least be able to pick and choose what you want. If a salad is available, give yourself a generous portion. Next, choose the vegetable, unless it's covered in butter or a sauce. Baked potatoes, of course, are fine. If the main dish is simply too fattening, either take just a small amount or leave it altogether. Remember, you don't have to eat everything that's available.

If there's no buffet, and you're simply served a prepared meal, do the best you can. Chicken, fish, beef, pasta, vegetables, potatoes, and fruit are your basic foods. Eat those if they're served. Avoid casseroles or dishes with sauces. It's okay to leave foods you should not have. After all, losing weight and changing your metabolism are serious matters. It's a little like treating yourself for a disease—the disease of *metabolic suppression.* So don't take it lightly. If you don't stick to the diet as closely as possible day after day, you'll simply be slowing your progress. I'm sure you don't want your weight loss to take any longer than is necessary.

If the host and hostess are close friends or relatives, you may want to let them know about your diet when you accept the invitation. In most cases, they'll surely try to give you what you need.

Once you arrive at the dinner party, you must be able to refuse offers of certain foods that are definitely off limits. Say "no" to the wine, and "no" to dessert, unless it's fruit, of course. You're not going to hurt anyone's feelings. Whether you realize it or not, most of your friends couldn't care less what you eat. And no one is going to tempt you, especially if they know you're on the New Hilton Head Metabolism Diet. Be gracious but firm. Say, "No, thank you. I don't care for dessert, but I would like a cup of that great coffee of yours. By the way, Flo, that meal was delicious."

One final word about dinner parties: I have found that increasing your exercise the day before, the day of, and the day after the party has a tremendous impact on your commitment and resolve. Try to exercise after *three* meals each day instead of only two. That way, should you eat a few extra calories, they'll be burned off quickly and won't affect your progress.

TRAVELING FOR BUSINESS OR PLEASURE

Whether you're on a vacation or a business trip, you can still follow the New Hilton Head Metabolism Diet.

The first problem arises during the course of travel by plane or auto. If you're flying, find out in advance if a meal will be served on the airplane. If so, call and arrange for a special meal. This is a routine procedure; the airlines are used to it. While they won't prepare different individual menus, they will serve a low-calorie meal. Ask for either the low-calorie meal, the diabetic meal, the low-sodium meal, or the vegetarian meal. All of these are nutritionally well-balanced and low in calories. In fact, these meals are always more appetizing and attractively served than the regular meals everyone else gets. Be sure to order your special food ahead of time, when you make your reservation, or they probably won't be able to accommodate you.

If your flight is just a short hop or a series of short hops, try to arrange your schedule so that you eat before you leave and upon your arrival. If you end up eating in an airport, avoid the little snack and hot dog stands; take the time to go to the larger, more varied cafeteria-style restaurants most airports have. If you're eating lunch, choose a salad or fruit plate. For dinner, chicken is standard cafeteria fare and a good choice, unless it's fried or smothered in sauce. If nothing looks appropriate, have a salad or fruit plate for dinner, then make up the calories at your minimeal.

If you're really pressed for time, buy a piece of fruit and eat it as your minimeal. Then eat your lunch or dinner when you have the opportunity. You might even bring fruit with you from home, so you'll be prepared.

And don't just sit around the airport. Have your meal, whether large or small, and get walking. Airports can be a great place to walk. Just keep yourself moving while you're waiting for the plane. Most passengers sit or stand for an hour or more, feeling bored and wasting time. You can be stirring up your metabolism, taking advantage of the extra time to burn more calories. There's a regular traveler in the Atlanta airport who takes along his jogging clothes, changes in the restroom, and runs while waiting for his next connection.

If you're traveling by car, plan your trip carefully. Try to allow enough time for meals. If you're rushed to get where you're going, you won't take the time to eat properly. Take a picnic meal with you if you are in a big hurry. Most of my meals can be prepared ahead of time and taken along in the car. If you'll be eating at a roadside restaurant, avoid the fast food places. Try to find a family restaurant that could serve you at least an approximation of your diet meals. It might take a little more time, but isn't your weight problem worth it? If a fast food restaurant is all that's available, choose one with a salad bar.

When you're taking a meal with you in the car, make sure you take *only* that meal. Some families get into the habit of loading the car with snack foods, even if the destination is only two or three hours away. This sets a bad precedent for all concerned. And don't eat your diet meal whenever you feel hungry. Set a definite mealtime, stop the car, and take time to eat. If you're near a park or highway rest area, you may even be able to take a twenty-minute walk. This would allow you to stretch and also serve as your after-meal Thermal Walk.

Once you arrive at your destination, follow my menu plan whether you're preparing your own meals or eating out in restaurants. If, for example, you're staying with friends for the weekend, let them know about your diet ahead of time. They don't have to change their meal plans completely, but if they're friends, they'll certainly want to help you out. Also, make certain you continue with the exercise plan. This is especially important when you are away from home and your routine is disrupted.

BUSINESS AND SOCIAL MEALS

In the course of dieting, you may have to attend a business lunch or dinner or a club luncheon. I'm talking about those already prepared meals where everyone gets the same thing. Creamed chicken is definitely not on the New Hilton Head Metabolism Diet. You basically have three choices on these occasions.

First, you could eat before or after the meal and just enjoy the meeting or the company of others without eating the prepared meal. Second, you could eat the salad and fruit, if available, as your minimeal and eat again later. Third, you could try to get by with the meal if it happens to be steak, plain chicken, or roast beef. Just pick and choose and trim off any excess fat. Eat the salad, the entree, and the vegetable; skip the dessert.

Chapter 17

◼ ◼ ◼

SUBSTITUTIONS

To provide a little more flexibility on the diet, I'm giving you a list of substitutes for the fruits, vegetables, and protein foods on my menus. Keep in mind that the closer you stick to my menu plans, the better you'll do—and the faster you'll lose weight. But I do realize that some vegetables and fruits are easier to buy at certain times of the year. Since I strongly advise fresh fruits and vegetables, you'll need to know about substitutions as the seasons vary. I also realize that you may have allergies or strong likes or dislikes to take into account.

FRUITS

My menus often call for fruit, especially at breakfast. You can substitute any of the following fruits for one another in the same portion. One piece of any of the following is approximately equal in calories.

Apple	Pear
Banana	Orange
Grapefruit	Nectarine
	Tangerine

Other fruits vary in their calorie counts. To make substitutions easy for you, the following list gives you the portions of different fruits that are equal to a half piece of any of the above fruits. You can substitute any of these fruits for one another or for the above list, as long as you use the portion indicated.

Apricots	2 whole
Blackberries	1/2 cup
Blueberries	1/2 cup
Raspberries	1/2 cup
Strawberries	3/4 cup
Fig	1 whole
Grapes	3/4 cup
Mango	1 whole
Cantaloupe	1/4
Honeydew	1/8
Watermelon	1 cup
Papaya	3/4
Peach	1 whole
Persimmon	1 whole
Pineapple	1/2 cup
Plums	2 whole
Prunes	2 whole
Raisins	1 1/2 tablespoons

VEGETABLES

The following are what I call the Group I vegetables. One half (1/2) cup of any of these can be substituted for any other. So, if my menu calls for green beans or asparagus, you can substitute any of the following, as long as it's the same portion.

Asparagus	Okra
Green beans	Summer squash

Broccoli	Carrots
Brussels sprouts	Rhubarb
Cauliflower	Tomatoes
Cabbage	Turnips
Eggplant	Kale
Collard greens	Turnip greens
Mustard greens	Zucchini
Spinach	Beets

The following are my Group II vegetables. These contain about three times as many calories as the Group I vegetables. They each can be substituted for one another, but *never* substitute a Group I vegetable for a Group II vegetable. However, you can substitute in the other direction. If your menu calls for corn on the cob, you can substitute 1 1/2 cups of a Group I vegetable. (You can have three times as much of a Group I vegetable).

Corn	Peas
Corn on the cob	Parsnips
Lima beans	

PROTEIN FOODS

Because of strong likes or dislikes or allergies, you may have to substitute one protein food for another. I suggest you avoid any substitutions of this type unless you have a definite allergy, or get physically ill from eating certain foods. Make sure you follow my portions when you substitute, so you keep the calories the same.

Beef	1 ounce
Lamb	1 ounce
Veal	1 ounce

Chicken (without skin)	1 ounce
Turkey (without skin)	1 ounce
Cornish hen (without skin)	1 ounce
Fish	1 1/2 ounces
Cottage cheese (low-fat)	1/4 cup
Egg	1 whole (small)

Remember, however, certain protein foods—beef, for example—contain more fat, and by substituting you will be throwing off the nutritional balance of the diet.

LIKES, DISLIKES, AND ALLERGIES

Avoid changes in my basic menu plans. If you dislike vegetables, learn to like them. Before you resist a food, give yourself a fighting chance. Try just a little of foods that are not your favorites. I've included such a variety of normal, everyday foods that almost everybody can stick to the New Hilton Head Metabolism Diet easily.

If you have food allergies, you might want to go over the diet with your physician or allergist. Let him or her guide and supervise you in making any substitutions.

Chapter 18
◪ ◪ ◪

THE NEW HILTON HEAD METABOLISM DIET RECIPES

These recipes provide variety during any stage of the diet. All of them were developed and tested at the Hilton Head Health Institute and have received rave reviews.

Pasta

◪ BAKED ZITI

Yield: 4 servings	Serving size: 1 1/2 cups
290 cal/serving 3.74g fat	% cal fat: 11%
carbo: 71%	protein: 18%

INGREDIENTS:

8 ounces dry ziti noodles (4 cups cooked)
1/2 teaspoon ground nutmeg
1 tablespoon chopped fresh parsley
1 tablespoon part-skim ricotta cheese
2 cups tomato sauce
4 tablespoons grated part-skim mozzarella cheese

PROCEDURE:

1. Preheat oven to 400°

2. Prepare ziti noodles
3. Drain noodles and add nutmeg, parsley, and ricotta cheese
4. Place 1 cup ziti mixture in each of four oven-proof bowls; top with 1/2 cup tomato sauce, sprinkle with 1 tablespoon mozzarella cheese
5. Bake until cheese is lightly browned, approximately 15 minutes

🖾 Cheese Filled Manicotta

Yield: 4 servings	Serving size: 1 manicotta
340 cal/serving 6.25g fat	% cal fat: 16%
carbo: 63%	protein: 21%

INGREDIENTS:

4 manicotta
10 tablespoons part-skim ricotta cheese
2 medium egg whites
4 tablespoons grated Parmesan cheese
4 tablespoons chopped fresh parsley
nutmeg (optional)
2 cups tomato sauce

PROCEDURE:

1. Preheat oven to 400°
2. Parboil manicotta for 6 minutes
3. Mix together ricotta cheese, egg whites, Parmesan cheese, parsley, and nutmeg
4. Fill each manicotta with cheese mixture, place in baking dish, cover with tomato sauce, and bake for 30 minutes

▧ FETTUCINI ALFREDO

Yield: 4 servings	Serving size: 1 cup
250 cal/serving 2.96g fat	% cal fat: 11%
carbo: 72%	protein: 17%

INGREDIENTS:

1/2 pound dry fettucini
1 teaspoon corn-oil margarine (low fat)
1 tablespoon skim milk
3 tablespoons plain low-fat yogurt
1 egg white
freshly ground black pepper
2 tablespoons grated Parmesan cheese

PROCEDURE:

1. Cook fettucini al dente
2. Place margarine in chafing dish
3. Add fettucini and toss gently till margarine has mixed with noodles
4. In separate bowl mix well skim milk and yogurt; add to fettucini and toss
5. Add egg white, pepper, grated cheese, and toss once again

◘ GNOCCHI

Yield: 6 servings	*Serving size: 1 cup*
260 cal/serving 2g fat	*% cal fat: 7%*
carbo: 76%	protein: 17%

INGREDIENTS:

2 cups mashed potatoes (fresh or instant, no added milk or butter)

1/2 cup egg whites or egg substitute

3 cups flour

vegetable spray

1/4 cup grated Parmesan cheese

PROCEDURE:

1. If using instant potatoes, boil 1 cup skim milk and 1 cup water and stir in potato flakes (or follow directions)
2. Place mashed potatoes and egg whites in a bowl and mix together
3. Gradually knead in flour (you may use a mixer with dough hooks) until you form a dough ball (you may not need to use all the flour)
4. Using the excess flour, roll the dough into 1/2 inch diameter tubes and cut into 1-inch lengths
5. Fill a medium saucepan approximately 1/2 full with water; bring water to a boil and drop in the dough pieces
6. Boil for 6–8 minutes, stirring occasionally, then drain
7. Spray a cookie sheet with vegetable spray and place the gnocchi on the sheet
8. Sprinkle with Parmesan or low-fat cheese of your choice and broil until golden (may also be served with tomato sauce)

◼ HOT PASTA PRIMAVERA

Yield: 4 servings	Serving size: 2 cups
300 cal/serving 5.17g fat	% cal fat: 15%
carbo: 63%	protein: 22%

INGREDIENTS:

6 ounces dry linguini or fettucini noodles
1/2 cup diced zucchini
1/2 cup diced summer squash
1/2 cup diced green beans
1/2 cup diced carrots
1/2 cup diced broccoli
1/2 cup diced onions
1 teaspoon minced garlic
2 teaspoons olive oil
1 1/2 cups evaporated skim milk
1/4 cup grated Parmesan cheese
black pepper to taste

PROCEDURE:

1. Cook pasta al dente
2. Heat medium-sized skillet and sauté vegetables and garlic in olive oil until tender
3. Add evaporated skim milk to vegetables and bring back to a simmer
4. When mixture begins to thicken add fettucini and cheese and toss with vegetables, remove from stove and serve immediately

◼ Lasagna

Yield: 12 servings	Serving size: 3" x 3" square or 1 1/2 cups
270 cal/serving 4.96g fat carbo: 56%	% cal fat: 16% protein: 28%

INGREDIENTS:

1 pound dry lasagna noodles
4 cups diced unpeeled zucchini
1 cup thinly sliced mushrooms
4 cups tomato sauce
3 cups low-fat cottage cheese
1 cup shredded part-skim mozzarella
4 tablespoons grated Parmesan cheese

PROCEDURE:

1. Cook lasagna noodles until chewy (about three-quarters done); drain and cool
2. Place one-third of noodles, slightly overlapping, in bottom of 10 x 13 x 2 baking dish
3. Proceed to layer ingredients evenly in the following order:
   - Zucchini and mushrooms
   - 2 1/2 cups tomato sauce
   - Another third of noodles
   - 3 cups cottage cheese
   - Mozzarella cheese
   - Remaining third of noodles
   - Remaining 1 1/2 cups tomato sauce
   - Parmesan cheese
4. Cover with aluminum foil and bake at 400° for 1/2 hour; uncover and bake for additional 1/2 hour

NOTE: Lasagna will be firmer and more flavorful if prepared, cooled, and reheated.

▧ MACARONI & CHEESE #1

Yield: 4 servings	Serving size: 1 cup
200 cal/serving 3.1g fat	% cal fat: 14%
carbo: 50%	protein: 36%

INGREDIENTS:

1 cup dry (2 cups cooked) elbow macaroni
1 1/2 cups low-fat cottage cheese
1/2 cup skim milk
2 tablespoons grated Parmesan cheese

PROCEDURE:

1. Preheat oven to 400°
2. Cook macaroni and rinse
3. Using blender, cream together cottage cheese and milk
4. Combine macaroni and cheese sauce in baking dish
5. Sprinkle with Parmesan cheese
6. Bake for 1/2 hour

▧ MACARONI & CHEESE #2

Yield: 8 servings	Serving size: 1 1/4 cups
281 cal/serving 3g fat	% cal fat: 10%
carbo: 66%	protein: 24%

INGREDIENTS:

1 pound dry elbow macaroni
3/4 cup low-fat cottage cheese
1/4 cup skim milk
4 ounces light Velveeta cheese

PROCEDURE:

1. In a large saucepan of boiling water add the macaroni and boil for 8–10 minutes, stirring occasionally to prevent sticking
2. Blend the cottage cheese and milk in a blender until smooth
3. Pour the cottage cheese mixture in a small saucepan and heat on medium-low
4. Dice the Velveeta and stir into cottage cheese mixture until cheeses are blended
5. Drain pasta and pour back into saucepan
6. Add cheese sauce and stir into pasta
7. Serve immediately

N PASTA & VEGGIES #1

Yield: 4 servings	*Serving size: 3 cups*
365 cal/serving 10.4g fat	*% cal fat: 25%*
carbo: 54%	*protein: 21%*

INGREDIENTS:

6 ounces dry pasta (3/4 cup cooked per person)
2 cups sliced mushrooms
2 cups sliced carrots
2 cups diced broccoli
2 cups plain nonfat yogurt
8 tablespoons grated Parmesan cheese
4 tablespoons low-fat corn-oil margarine

PROCEDURE:

1. Cook pasta al dente and drain
2. Steam vegetables for 10 minutes

3. In small saucepan heat yogurt, Parmesan cheese, and margarine; do not boil or yogurt will separate
4. Toss vegetables and pasta together
5. Place in bowl and pour sauce over
6. Serve while hot

🔖 PASTA & VEGGIES #2

Yield: 4 servings	Serving size: 3 cups
385 cal/serving 12.3g fat	% cal fat: 29%
carbo: 58%	protein: 13%

INGREDIENTS:

6 ounces dry pasta
8 tablespoons olive oil
2 cups sliced mushrooms
2 cups sliced yellow squash
2 cups sliced zucchini
2 cups sliced onions
4 cloves minced garlic
4 tablespoons grated Parmesan cheese

PROCEDURE:

1. Cook pasta al dente
2. In 1 teaspoon olive oil sauté vegetables and garlic until tender
3. Toss pasta with remaining oil
4. Pour vegetables over pasta
5. Sprinkle Parmesan cheese; garnish with tomato wedge; serve hot

◪ Spaghetti

Yield: 4 servings	*Serving size: 1 1/4 cups*
210 cal/serving 2.78g fat	*% cal fat: 12%*
carbo: 71%	*protein: 17%*

INGREDIENTS:

3 cups cooked spaghetti noodles

2 cups tomato sauce (use recipe on p. 227 or a commercial variety)

4 tablespoons grated Parmesan cheese

PROCEDURE:

1. Pour heated tomato sauce over drained spaghetti
2. Sprinkle with Parmesan cheese and serve immediately

◪ Stuffed Shells

Yield: 4 servings	*Serving size: 3 shells*
300 cal/serving 6.44g fat	*% cal fat: 19%*
carbo: 55%	*protein: 26%*

INGREDIENTS:

12 jumbo pasta shells

2 cups chopped broccoli

1/2 cup low-fat cottage cheese

2 1/2 ounces shredded part-skim mozzarella cheese

1/4 cup grated Parmesan cheese

1/4 cup skim milk

1/4 teaspoon dried oregano

1/8 teaspoon white pepper

1 cup tomato sauce

PROCEDURE:

1. Preheat oven to 375°
2. Boil shells until chewy; rinse and cool
3. Steam broccoli for 5 minutes; set aside
4. Place cottage cheese, mozzarella, Parmesan, and milk in blender and blend until smooth
5. Combine blended cheeses, spices, and broccoli in bowl and mix well
6. Stuff shells and place in casserole dish (10 x 13 x 2)
7. Pour tomato sauce over shells and bake for 20 minutes; serve immediately

N TUNA-MUSHROOM CASSEROLE

Yield: 9 cups	Serving size: 1 cup
200 cal/serving 7.7g fat	% cal fat: 15%
carbo: 54%	protein: 22%

INGREDIENTS:

1/2 cup diced onion
2 cups sliced mushrooms
2 cups skim milk
1 cup white wine
1/2 cup flour dissolved in 1 cup water
4 cups cooked noodles or shells (2 cups uncooked)
8 ounces drained water-packed tuna
white pepper to taste

PROCEDURE:

1. Preheat oven to 400°
2. In nonstick fry pan, sauté onions and mushrooms until tender

3. Place milk and wine in sauce pan and heat on medium heat
4. When milk bubbles, add flour paste and whisk constantly until blended
5. Simmer for 5 minutes, stirring constantly; remove from stove
6. Mix in cooked noodles, onions, mushrooms, pepper, and tuna
7. Pour into a small casserole dish and bake 25–30 minutes
8. Serve immediately

◪ Vermicelli Sciacca

Yield: 4 servings	Serving size: 1 1/4 cups
300 cal/serving 7.7g fat	% cal fat: 23%
carbo: 59%	protein: 18%

INGREDIENTS:

1/2 pound vermicelli
2 tablespoons low-fat corn-oil margarine
4 ounces part-skim ricotta cheese
2 tablespoons freshly chopped parsley
4 tablespoons grated Parmesan cheese
black pepper to taste

PROCEDURE:

1. Cook vermicelli al dente
2. Drain and place in warm bowl with 1 tablespoon margarine
3. Melt 1 tablespoon margarine in sauce pan
4. Stir in ricotta and stir until smooth

5. Pour over vermicelli
6. Sprinkle with parsley, Parmesan, and pepper
7. Toss and serve

Pizza

⬛ PITA PIZZA

Yield: 4 servings	Serving size: 1 pita
220 cal/serving 2.31g fat	% cal fat: 9%
carbo: 74%	protein: 17%

INGREDIENTS:

8 ounces tomato sauce
4 whole wheat pitas
2 cups sautéed mushrooms, Julienne-style cut onions and peppers
4 tablespoons (1 ounce) shredded part-skim mozzarella cheese

PROCEDURE:

1. Preheat oven to 450°
2. Spread tomato sauce over each pita bread
3. Sprinkle mushrooms, onions, and peppers over sauce
4. Sprinkle cheese over vegetables
5. Place on cookie sheet and bake until cheese bubbles, approximately 10 minutes; serve immediately

Poultry

▧ CATALINA CHICKEN

Yield: 4 servings	Serving size: 1 breast
150 cal/serving 2.36g fat	% cal fat: 14%
carbo: 11%	protein: 75%

INGREDIENTS:

4 (4-ounce) skinless, boneless chicken breasts
4 tablespoons low-fat Catalina salad dressing
1 teaspoon dried basil

PROCEDURE:

1. Preheat oven to 400°
2. Place chicken breasts in a small oven pan and cover
   with Catalina and basil
3. Bake for 10–12 minutes or until cooked thoroughly;
   serve immediately

▧ CHICKEN A LA KING

Yield: 4 servings	*Serving size: 1 1/2 cups*
235 cal/serving 10.1g fat	*% cal fat: 39%*
carbo: 13%	*protein: 48%*

INGREDIENTS:

1 pound diced skinless, boneless chicken breast (1/2 inch pieces)

2 1/2 cups water

3 tablespoons flour

3 teaspoons low-fat corn-oil margarine

1/2 cup sliced mushrooms

1/2 cup diced pimento

1/2 cup diced green pepper

1/2 cup diced onions

PROCEDURE:

1. Poach chicken in simmering water for 10 minutes (uncovered)
2. Combine flour and margarine to form a roux; in separate pan, cook over medium heat for 5 minutes, stirring constantly
3. Add vegetables to chicken, then add roux
4. Cook for 10 minutes, stirring occasionally and serve immediately
5. Serve over rice, if desired (calories for rice not included)

N Chicken Cacciatore

Yield: 4 servings	Serving size: 1 breast
280 cal/serving 6.44g fat	% cal fat: 21%
carbo: 26%	protein: 43%

INGREDIENTS:

4 (4-ounce) boneless, skinless chicken breasts
1 cup sliced mushrooms
1 cup minced onion
1 cup diced bell pepper
1 cup burgundy wine
2 cups tomato sauce (commercially prepared or use
recipe on page 227)

PROCEDURE:

1. Combine all ingredients in a skillet and simmer for
   20–30 minutes, covered
2. Place chicken on plate and pour hot sauce and
   vegetables over chicken
3. Serve with your favorite pasta (calories not included,
   add 100 calories for 1/2 cup)

◪ CHICKEN CORDON BLEU

Yield: 4 servings	Serving size: 1 breast
545 cal/serving 16g fat	% cal fat: 27%
carbo: 24%	protein: 49%

INGREDIENTS:

4 (5-ounce) boneless, skinless chicken breasts
2 tablespoons Dijon mustard
4 (1-ounce) slices Swiss cheese
4 ounces low-sodium, low-fat shaved baked ham
1/2 cup all-purpose flour
1/2 cup egg substitute or egg whites, beaten with whisk
1 cup Italian bread crumbs
vegetable spray

PROCEDURE:

1. Preheat oven to 400°
2. Place chicken breasts (smooth side down) on a cutting board and cover with clear plastic wrap
3. Pound each breast until doubled in size; remove plastic
4. Brush each breast with mustard
5. Place 1 slice low-fat Swiss cheese on each breast, then sprinkle ham over the cheese
6. Starting at narrow end of breast, roll up, tucking in the ends as you roll
7. Hold together and dip in flour, then eggs, then bread crumbs
8. Spray a baking pan with vegetable spray and place the breasts on it
9. Bake in oven for 20–25 minutes or until golden brown

Chicken En Croute

Yield: 4 servings	Serving size: 1 breast
153 cal/serving 2.26g fat	% cal fat: 15%
carbo: 17%	protein: 68%

INGREDIENTS:

1 cup steamed spinach
1/2 cup evaporated skim milk
pinch ground ginger
pinch ground nutmeg
4 phyllo leaves
4 (2-ounce) boneless, skinless chicken breasts, cooked
1 egg white, beaten

PROCEDURE:

1. Preheat oven to 375°
2. Drain spinach well, using your hands to squeeze out excess water
3. Add evaporated milk, ginger and nutmeg
4. Open phyllo leaves and place one chicken breast in one corner of each
5. Place spinach mixture on top of chicken; fold phyllo over chicken and spinach and form a square package
6. Brush package with egg white
7. Bake on cookie sheet for approximately 10–15 minutes and serve immediately

◼ CHICKEN PARMESAN

Yield: 4 servings	Serving size: 1 breast
275 cal/serving 6.36g fat	% cal fat: 21%
carbo: 10%	protein: 69%

INGREDIENTS:

vegetable spray

4 (4-ounce) skinless, boneless chicken breasts

1 cup tomato sauce (commercially prepared or use recipe on page 227)

4 ounces part-skim mozzarella cheese

PROCEDURE:

1. Spray small skillet with vegetable spray
2. Place chicken in skillet and cover with tomato sauce
3. Place 1 ounce of cheese on each chicken breast
4. Simmer covered for 10 minutes; serve immediately

◪ Chicken Tetrazzini

Yield: 6 servings	Serving size: 1 3/4 cups
160 cal/serving 2.46g fat	% cal fat: 14%
carbo: 32%	protein: 54%

INGREDIENTS:

6 ounces dry pasta
3 cups chicken stock
1/2 cup evaporated skim milk
1 pound (1/2 inch diced pieces) raw chicken breasts
3 cups sliced mushrooms
1/2 cup all-purpose flour
3/4 cup water
1/4 cup sherry (optional)
pinch of white pepper

PROCEDURE:

1. Cook the pasta al dente and set aside
2. Combine chicken stock and evaporated milk in a heavy sauce pan and bring to a boil
3. Add chicken and cook for 20 minutes
4. Add mushrooms
5. Dissolve flour with water to make a thickener and add this to the chicken mixture
6. Add the sherry and white pepper
7. Serve 1 cup of the chicken mixture on 3/4 cup of pasta

◼ COQ AU VIN

Yield: 4 servings	Serving size: 1 breast
265 cal/serving 4.26g fat	% cal fat: 14%
carbo: 17%	protein: 40%

INGREDIENTS:

3 cups red burgundy wine
1 cup Julienne-style cut onion
1 bay leaf
1 teaspoon dried thyme
1 garlic clove
4 (4-ounce) boneless, skinless chicken breasts
2 cups mushroom caps
4 tablespoons cornstarch

PROCEDURE:

1. Place first five ingredients in small skillet
2. Bring ingredients to a boil, then reduce heat and simmer for 5 minutes
3. Add chicken and mushrooms and continue to simmer 8–10 minutes
4. Remove garlic clove and bay leaf
5. Dissolve cornstarch in 1/4 cup of water and stir into sauce
6. Place chicken on plate, pour sauce and vegetables over chicken; serve immediately

◨ Italian Chicken #1

Yield: 4 servings	Serving size: 1 breast
230 cal/serving 10.1g fat	% cal fat: 40%
carbo: 5%	protein: 55%

INGREDIENTS:

4 teaspoons olive oil
2 teaspoons garlic powder
2 teaspoons dried oregano
2 teaspoons dried basil
2 tablespoons water
4 (3-ounce) skinless, boneless chicken breasts
2 ounces shredded, part-skim mozzarella cheese

PROCEDURE:

1. Place oil, spices, and water in small skillet
2. Add chicken, cover and simmer for 15 minutes
3. Add cheese and continue to simmer uncovered until cheese has melted
4. Serve immediately

◼ ITALIAN CHICKEN #2

Yield: 4 servings	Serving size: 1 breast
250 cal/serving 4g fat	% cal fat: 29%
carbo: 7%	protein: 64%

INGREDIENTS:

1/2 cup low-fat Italian dressing
2 teaspoons garlic powder
2 teaspoons dried oregano
2 teaspoons dried basil
4 (4-ounce) skinless, boneless chicken breasts
2 tablespoons grated Parmesan cheese

PROCEDURE:

1. Place dressing and spices in small skillet; heat and add chicken
2. Sprinkle Parmesan cheese on top of chicken
3. Simmer covered for 15–20 minutes; serve immediately

▨ Jamaican Chicken

Yield: 4 servings	*Serving size:* 1 breast
200 cal/serving 4g fat	*% cal fat:* 10%
carbo: 28%	*protein:* 62%

INGREDIENTS:

4 (4-ounce) boneless, skinless chicken breasts
2 teaspoons instant coffee
2 tablespoons hot water
1/2 cup non-fat plain yogurt
4 pineapple slices

PROCEDURE:

1. Preheat oven to 350°
2. Place chicken in small baking dish
3. Dissolve coffee in hot water and stir it into the yogurt
4. Pour coffee yogurt over chicken and place pineapple on top
5. Bake for 30–40 minutes (may also be sautéed in small skillet); serve immediately

◼ LADY DAPHNE'S CHICKEN

Yield: 4 servings	Serving size: 1 breast
150 cal/serving 3.34g fat	% cal fat: 20%
carbo: 5%	protein: 75%

INGREDIENTS:

4 (3-ounce) skinless, boneless chicken breasts

4 tablespoons nonfat vanilla yogurt

2 teaspoons dried rosemary

PROCEDURE:

1. Preheat oven to 350°
2. Place chicken in ungreased baking pan and bake for 30 minutes
3. Remove from oven and cover with yogurt
4. Sprinkle top with rosemary
5. Return to oven for 15 minutes before serving

◼ QUICKY CHICKY BLUE

Yield: 4 servings	*Serving size:* 1 breast
240 cal/serving 7.63g fat	% cal fat: 29%
carbo: 6%	protein: 65%

INGREDIENTS:

4 (4-ounce) skinless, boneless chicken breasts
1/2 cup low-fat bleu cheese dressing
4 teaspoons freshly chopped parsley

PROCEDURE:

1. Place chicken in small skillet and add a little water
2. Pour bleu cheese dressing over chicken
3. Sprinkle with parsley
4. Simmer covered for 15–20 minutes; serve immediately

◪ STIR-FRY CHICKEN

Yield: 4 servings	Serving size: 1 3/4 cups
240 cal/serving 4.45g fat	% cal fat: 17%
carbo: 19%	protein: 64%

INGREDIENTS:

1 tablespoon canola oil
1 pound skinless, boneless chicken breasts, Julienne sliced
1 cup sliced mushrooms
1 cup diced broccoli
1/4 cup diced onion
1 cup pea pods
1 cup sliced yellow squash
1/2 cup sliced carrot
1/4 cup water
1 tablespoon cornstarch dissolved with 1/4 cup water
1 tablespoon low-sodium soy sauce

PROCEDURE:

1. Heat wok to medium heat (about 300°)
2. Add oil and chicken; stir-fry for 30 seconds
3. Raise heat to high; add all vegetables and water and stir-fry for 2 minutes
4. Add dissolved cornstarch and soy sauce
5. Stir-fry for 1 minute; serve immediately

◪ Tarragon Lime Chicken

Yield: 4 servings	Serving size: 1 breast
280 cal/serving 10.9g fat	% cal fat: 35%
carbo: 5%	protein: 51%

INGREDIENTS:

2 tablespoons canola oil
1/2 cup fresh lime juice
1/2 cup dry white wine
2 garlic cloves
2 tablespoons fresh chopped chives
1 tablespoon fresh chopped mint
1/2 teaspoon dried tarragon
1/2 teaspoon fresh ground pepper
1/4 teaspoon dry mustard
1/2 teaspoon Worcestershire sauce
4 (4-ounce) skinless, boneless chicken breasts (pounded lightly)

PROCEDURE:

1. Combine all ingredients except chicken in a bowl
2. Place chicken pieces in a baking dish
3. Pour marinade over chicken and marinate overnight
4. Broil chicken under broiler, brushing on marinade every minute until chicken is cooked, approximately 10 minutes; serve immediately

◫ TURKEY HASH

Yield: 4 servings
190 cal/serving 1.58g fat
carbo: 14%

Serving size: 1 3/4 cups
% cal fat: 7%
protein: 79%

INGREDIENTS:

1 1/2 cups chicken stock
1 pound diced cooked turkey breast (1/4" diced size)
1 cup chopped onions
1 1/2 cups chopped celery
1 cup chopped green pepper
1/2 teaspoon dried thyme

PROCEDURE:

1. Place all ingredients in pot
2. Cook on high heat for 5 minutes; reduce to low and
   cook 30 minutes, stirring occasionally
3. Serve immediately

Meat

▨ Beef Stew

Yield: 4 servings	Serving size: 3 cups
424 cal/serving 9g fat	% cal fat: 20%
carbo: 43%	protein: 37%

INGREDIENTS:

vegetable spray
1 cup diced medium onion
1 pound trimmed flank steak cut in 1/2-inch cubes
1 cup diced carrots
1 cup diced celery
1 cup sliced mushrooms
2 (8-ounce) diced potatoes
2 teaspoons Kitchen Bouquet browning and seasoning sauce
1 teaspoon salt (optional)
4 cups low-salt beef broth
1/2 cup flour plus 1/2 cup water

PROCEDURE:

1. In a medium sauce pan sprayed with vegetable spray, sauté the onions and steak for 10 minutes
2. Add the vegetables, potatoes, spices, and broth and simmer for 20 minutes
3. Whisk the flour and water mixture until smooth and slowly add to the meat and vegetables; simmer, stirring frequently, for 10 minutes
4. Serve immediately

BEEF STROGANOFF

Yield: 4 servings	Serving size: 1 3/4 cups
375 cal/serving 8.67g fat	% cal fat: 21%
carbo: 31%	protein: 46%

INGREDIENTS:

1 pound diced tenderloin or round steak (1/2" diced
pieces)
1/2 cup diced onions
1 clove garlic
1 cup sliced mushrooms
1 tablespoon tomato paste
pepper to taste
1/2 cup water
1/4 cup cooking sherry
1 cup nonfat plain yogurt
2 cups cooked egg noodles

PROCEDURE:

1. Sauté beef with onions and garlic
2. When beef is browned add mushrooms, tomato paste,
   pepper, water, and sherry; simmer for 5 minutes
3. Remove from heat and add yogurt
4. Serve over egg noodles

N Beef Kabob

Yield: 4 servings	Serving size: 1 skewer
240 cal/serving 6.75g fat	% cal fat: 25%
carbo: 17%	protein: 58%

INGREDIENTS:

1 pound beef, preferably round steak or tenderloin, cut in cubes (1" in size)
1 cup onion cut in quarters
1 green bell pepper cut in 8 pieces
4 cherry tomatoes

PROCEDURE:

1. Divide ingredients and arrange on 4 skewers
2. Broil until tender

*NOTE: You may substitute shrimp or chicken for the beef and supplement the vegetables with fruits such as pineapple, apples, pitted cherries, etc.

▧ CHINESE PEPPER STEAK

Yield: 4 servings	Serving size: 1 1/2 cups
284 cal/serving 6g fat	% cal fat: 19%
carbo: 26%	protein: 55%

INGREDIENTS:

1 pound trimmed round or flank steak
1/4 cup soy sauce
1 cup beef stock or bouillon
2 teaspoons granulated garlic
1 teaspoon onion powder
1/2 teaspoon ginger
2 teaspoons olive oil
1 cup hot water
3 tablespoons cornstarch dissolved in 1/4 cup cold water
1 green pepper cut Julienne style
1 red pepper cut Julienne style
1/2 cup water chestnuts (optional)

PROCEDURE:

1. Cut steak in 1/2-inch strips
2. Marinate steak in soy sauce, bouillon, garlic, onion powder, and ginger for at least 2 hours
3. Drain meat, reserving 1/2 cup marinade; dry meat strips on paper towels
4. In a large skillet or wok, sauté the steak in 2 teaspoons olive oil until browned
5. Add marinade and 1 cup hot water and simmer covered for 1/2 hour
6. Stir the dissolved cornstarch into the beef mixture
7. Add the peppers and simmer for 5–10 minutes or until thickened

◪ Lamb With Mint Sauce

Yield: 4 servings	Serving size: 2 chops
250 cal/serving 11g fat	% cal fat: 40%
carbo: 3%	protein:57%

INGREDIENTS:

1/2 cup chopped fresh mint
4 packages or 4 teaspoons artificial sweetener
1/2 cup white vinegar
8 lean lamb chops

PROCEDURE:

1. Preheat oven to 325°
2. Place mint, sweetener, and vinegar in small sauce pan; simmer for 5 minutes
3. Place chops in baking dish, cover with sauce
4. Bake for 1/2 hour or until chops are tender
5. Serve immediately

◪ MOM'S MEATLOAF

Yield: 4 servings	Serving size: 1 slice
260 cal/serving 16.1g fat	% cal fat: 48%
carbo: 5%	protein: 47%

INGREDIENTS:

1/2 cup diced onion
1/2 cup diced green pepper
1/2 teaspoon hot sauce
2 teaspoons dried oregano
1 teaspoon garlic powder
2 teaspoons black pepper
1 pound ground round
4 egg whites

PROCEDURE:

1. Preheat oven to 400°
2. Simmer onion, green pepper, and spices in 1/2 cup water in skillet until vegetables are tender
3. Combine vegetables with beef and egg whites; mix by hand
4. Place in small loaf pan or casserole dish
5. Bake for 20–30 minutes
6. Slice into 4 equal pieces and serve

N Veal Marsala

Yield: 4 servings	*Serving size: 1 patty*
185 cal/serving 4.98g fat	*% cal fat: 24%*
carbo: 10%	*protein: 54%*

INGREDIENTS:

2 cups beef stock
1 cup marsala wine
4 garlic cloves
1 teaspoon black pepper
4 shallots or small onions
2 teaspoons freshly chopped parsley
cornstarch
4 (3-ounce) ground veal patties
vegetable spray
1 cup thinly sliced mushrooms

PROCEDURE:

1. Make a heavy brown sauce by boiling the first 6 ingredients; add 2–3 teaspoons cornstarch to thicken
2. Sauté veal on each side in nonstick skillet coated with vegetable spray
3. Add brown sauce and mushrooms to veal and sauté for 1 minute
4. Place veal on plate and cover with mushroom sauce

▧ Veal Parmesan

Yield: 4 servings	Serving size: 1 slice
335 cal/serving 11.5g fat	% cal fat: 31%
carbo: 28%	protein: 41%

INGREDIENTS:

4 (3-ounce) trimmed, lean veal slices

2 egg whites

4 slices low-calorie whole wheat bread, dried and grated into crumbs

8 tablespoons all-purpose flour

1 tablespoon olive oil

1 cup tomato sauce (commercially prepared or use recipe on page 227)

2 ounces grated part-skim mozzarella cheese

PROCEDURE:

1. Pound veal until thin
2. Beat egg whites in a bowl
3. Place bread crumbs and flour in separate bowls
4. Dip each piece of veal in flour, egg whites, then bread crumbs
5. Heat skillet and add olive oil
6. Sauté veal on each side until golden brown
7. Place veal in casserole dish, cover with tomato sauce, and sprinkle with cheese
8. Broil until cheese bubbles; serve immediately

N Veal Picatta

Yield: 4 servings	Serving size: 1 steak
285 cal/serving 10.5g fat	% cal fat: 33%
carbo: 17%	protein: 50%

INGREDIENTS:

4 (4-ounce) boneless trimmed veal steaks
1/2 cup wheat flour
2 tablespoons freshly chopped parsley
4 teaspoons low-fat corn-oil margarine
juice of 1 lemon

PROCEDURE:

1. Pound each piece of veal until thin
2. Mix flour and parsley together and place on a plate
3. Melt margarine in nonstick skillet and add lemon juice
4. Dust each side of veal steaks with flour/parsley mixture
5. Sauté veal steaks till done and serve immediately

NOTE: May replace with skinless chicken breasts

◼ VEAL ROLLETTES

Yield: 4 servings	Serving size: 1 steak
140 cal/serving 5.09g fat	% cal fat: 33%
carbo: 4%	protein: 63%

INGREDIENTS:

4 (2-ounce) boneless trimmed veal steaks
2 slices low-fat American cheese
4 large asparagus spears
vegetable spray

PROCEDURE:

1. Preheat oven to 400°
2. Pound each piece of veal until thin
3. Place 1/2 slice cheese and 1 asparagus spear on each piece of veal
4. Roll up veal to form small bundle and secure with toothpick
5. Spray small oven pan with vegetable spray
6. Place veal rolls in pan with toothpick facing up
7. Bake for 12–18 minutes; serve immediately

Seafood

◪ BARBECUED SHRIMP

Yield: 4 servings	Serving size: 1 skewer
120 cal/serving 2.69g fat	% cal fat: 15%
carbo: 25%	protein: 60%

INGREDIENTS:

1 pound raw, peeled shrimp
1 8-ounce can pineapple chunks
barbecue sauce (see recipe p. 223)

PROCEDURE:

1. Alternate shrimp and pineapple chunks on 4 skewers
2. Brush with barbecue sauce
3. Grill on hot grill for a few minutes on each side, continually basting with sauce
4. Serve immediately

◨ BLACKENED FISH

Yield: 4 servings	Serving size: 1 filet
190 cal/serving 7.73g fat	% cal fat: 37%
carbo: 6%	protein: 57%

INGREDIENTS:

seasoning mix:

1 tablespoon paprika
1 teaspoon onion powder
1 teaspoon garlic powder
1 teaspoon cayenne pepper
1/2 teaspoon white pepper
1/2 teaspoon black pepper
1/2 teaspoon ground oregano
1/2 teaspoon ground thyme
2 tablespoons low-fat corn-oil margarine
4 (5-ounce) fish filets (redfish, pompano, or tilefish) 1/2-inch thick

PROCEDURE:

1. Sift together seasoning mix
2. Melt margarine
3. Heat a cast-iron skillet on high for 10 minutes or until the bottom turns white
4. Lightly coat the filets with the seasoning mix
5. Add melted margarine to skillet (be careful because the grease will splatter)
6. Add filets and fry 1–2 minutes on each side
7. Serve immediately

◧ BREADED BAKED FISH FILETS

Yield: 4 servings	Serving size: 1 filet
426 cal/serving 8g fat	% cal fat: 17%
carbo: 42%	protein: 41%

INGREDIENTS:

4 egg whites
1 cup all-purpose flour
4 (6-ounce) fresh catfish (or any other thin white fish)
filets
1 cup seasoned bread crumbs
vegetable spray

PROCEDURE:

1. Preheat oven to 400°
2. Beat egg whites in a medium bowl
3. Lightly flour fish filets
4. Place filets in egg whites, then coat with bread crumbs
5. Spray a baking pan with vegetable spray
6. Place filets on pan and bake for 15–20 minutes, or
   until golden brown
7. Serve with low-fat tartar sauce (commercially
   prepared)

▧ FISH CREOLE

Yield: 4 servings	*Serving size: 1 filet*
215 cal/serving 7.63g fat	*% cal fat: 32%*
carbo: 17%	*protein: 51%*

INGREDIENTS:

4 cups diced tomatoes
1/2 cup diced green pepper
1/2 cup diced green onion or 1/4 cup diced shallots
2 cloves minced garlic
1 bay leaf
1 teaspoon olive oil
juice of 1 whole lemon
4 (5-ounce) fish filets

PROCEDURE:

1. Sauté vegetables, garlic, and bay leaf in olive oil until tender; set aside
2. Sprinkle lemon juice on fish; bake at 375° for 15 minutes
3. Place fish on plates and cover with vegetables; serve immediately

◫ Fish Parmesan

Yield: 4 servings	Serving size: 1 filet
275 cal/serving 11.4g fat	% cal fat: 37%
carbo: 7%	protein: 56%

INGREDIENTS:

4 (6-ounce) filets of flounder or other white fish
4 tablespoons grated onion
1 teaspoon dried oregano
1 teaspoon dried sweet basil
1/2 teaspoon fresh ground pepper
8 tablespoons grated Parmesan cheese
8 tablespoons lemon juice
4 tablespoons low-fat corn-oil margarine

PROCEDURE:

1. Place flounder on baking pan
2. Sprinkle onion, herbs, spices, and Parmesan cheese on fish
3. Cover all with lemon juice
4. Dot with margarine
5. Broil 8–10 minutes or until flaky; serve immediately

◫ Flounder With Dill Sauce

Yield: 4 servings	Serving size: 1 filet
120 cal/serving 1.79g fat	% cal fat: 13%
carbo: 8%	protein: 79%

INGREDIENTS:

4 (4-ounce) fresh flounder filets
8 tablespoons dill sauce (see recipe p. 224)

PROCEDURE:

1. Slowly heat dill sauce
2. Broil fish 5–8 minutes until flaky
3. Cover fish with sauce and serve immediately

◪ FLOUNDER WITH LEMON MARGARINE

Yield: 4 servings	*Serving size: 1 filet*
140 cal/serving 5.14g fat	*% cal fat: 33%*
carbo: 4%	*protein: 63%*

INGREDIENTS:

4 teaspoons low-fat corn-oil margarine
juice of 2 fresh lemons
vegetable spray
4 (4-ounce) flounder filets

PROCEDURE:

1. Preheat oven to 400°
2. Melt margarine in sauce pan; add lemon juice to margarine; set aside
3. Spray baking pan with vegetable spray
4. Place fish in pan; cover with sauce and bake 5–8 minutes or until flaky
5. Serve immediately

◐ Marinated Grilled Fish

Yield: 4 servings	Serving size: 1 steak
155 cal/serving 3.17g fat	% cal fat: 18%
carbo: 6%	protein: 76%

INGREDIENTS:

1/4 cup low-sodium soy sauce
1/4 cup low-fat Italian dressing
4 (5-ounce) fish steaks (use grouper, mahi-mahi, swordfish, or any thick filet)

PROCEDURE:

1. Mix soy sauce and dressing in a small bowl; pour over fish, cover, and refrigerate overnight
2. Grill fish on charcoal or gas grill about 5 minutes on each side; serve immediately

▧ SALMON PATTIES

Yield: 5 patties	Serving size: 1 patty
210 cal/serving 7.52g fat	% cal fat: 32%
carbo: 12%	protein: 56%

INGREDIENTS:

1 pound poached, drained salmon
3 slices low-calorie whole wheat bread
1/3 cup low-fat cottage cheese
2 tablespoons skim milk
1 tablespoon capers
1 tablespoon all-purpose flour

PROCEDURE:

1. Preheat oven to 400°
2. Prepare the salmon; after draining, flake the salmon in a bowl
3. Grate the bread into bread crumbs and set aside
4. Blend cottage cheese in a blender until smooth; add to the salmon
5. Add remaining ingredients except bread crumbs and mix thoroughly
6. Form salmon mixture into 5 patties, approximately 1/4 cup each
7. Place each patty in bread crumbs; coat each side
8. Place on a nonstick baking pan and bake for 8–10 minutes; serve immediately

▧ Shrimp Curry

Yield: 4 servings	*Serving size:* 1 cup
235 cal/serving 4.8g fat	*% cal fat:* 18%
carbo: 23%	*protein:* 59%

INGREDIENTS:

3 tablespoons flour
3 teaspoons low-fat corn-oil margarine
1/4 cup Chablis
1 diced pineapple ring
1/3 diced ripe banana
1 tablespoon minced onion
1 teaspoon curry powder
1/2 teaspoon mace powder
1/2 teaspoon dried thyme
1 bay leaf
2/3 cup skim milk
20 ounces cooked shrimp

PROCEDURE:

1. Combine flour and margarine to form a roux; set aside
2. In sauce pan heat wine, fruit, onion, and spices
3. Simmer for 5 minutes
4. Add milk and bring to simmer
5. Add roux and blend thoroughly
6. Bring back to simmer, stirring constantly
7. Add shrimp and stir for 1 minute
8. Serve over rice if desired (calories for rice not included)

▧ SHRIMP SCAMPI

Yield: 4 servings	Serving size: 3/4 cup
215 cal/serving 5.91g fat	% cal fat: 25%
carbo: 15%	protein: 60%

INGREDIENTS:

20 ounces cooked and peeled large shrimp
4 teaspoons low-fat corn-oil margarine
4 cloves garlic
2 slices finely grated low-calorie bread

PROCEDURE:

1. Slice shrimp halfway up the back, toward the tail
2. Place shrimp on baking sheet so that tails are facing upward
3. Melt margarine and squeeze garlic into it
4. Add bread to margarine and mix thoroughly
5. Pour mixture over shrimp and broil for 2–3 minutes; serve immediately

◨ Stir-Fry Shrimp (or Chicken)

Yield: 4 servings	Serving size: 2 1/2 cups
180 cal/serving 2.38g fat	% cal fat: 12%
carbo: 50%	protein: 38%

INGREDIENTS:

1 cup chicken stock (commercially prepared or use recipe on p. 229)

1/2 tablespoon fresh grated ginger

1/2 tablespoon fresh grated garlic

8 ounces shrimp (or 6 ounces chicken breast cut in bite-size pieces)

1 cup diced broccoli

1 cup Julienne-cut red peppers

1 cup Julienne-cut green peppers

1 cup diced scallions

1 cup fresh bean sprouts

1 cup sliced water chestnuts

1 cup pea pods

1 cup diced celery

1 tablespoon cornstarch or tapioca starch

1 tablespoon low-sodium soy sauce

PROCEDURE:

1. Heat wok on high
2. Add 3/4 cup chicken stock, ginger and garlic (if using chicken, add now and cook thoroughly)
3. Add vegetables and shrimp and stir for 2 minutes
4. Dissolve cornstarch or tapioca starch in 1/4 cup of chicken stock and add to stir-fry
5. Add soy sauce and serve immediately

▨ STUFFED FLOUNDER

Yield: 4 servings	*Serving size: 1 filet*
250 cal/serving 6.52g fat	*% cal fat: 23%*
carbo: 0%	*protein: 77%*

INGREDIENTS:

4 (5-ounce) filets of flounder or any other white fish

12 ounces fresh or frozen crabmeat

4 teaspoons low-fat corn-oil margarine

PROCEDURE:

1. Cut filets in half; place 4 halves in baking dish
2. Place crabmeat on fish in dish
3. Slice remaining pieces of fish in two lengthwise strips
4. Place these pieces on each side of crabmeat
5. Pour melted margarine over crabmeat and flounder
6. Put 1–2 tablespoons water in bottom of dish
7. Broil or bake until fish turns white (if baking, bake at 475° for 10 minutes)
8. Serve immediately

Salads

◾ Chicken Salad

Yield: 4 servings	Serving size: 1 tomato or 3/4 cup (when used for sandwich)
200 cal/serving 3.79g fat carbo: 45%	% cal fat: 17% protein: 39%

INGREDIENTS:

4 (2-ounce) cooked chicken breasts, diced
1 cup diced apple
1 cup diced celery
1/2 cup diced onion
4 tablespoons low-fat mayonnaise
4 whole medium tomatoes

PROCEDURE:

1. Place chicken, apple, celery, and onion in mixing bowl
2. Add mayonnaise and toss gently
3. Slice the tomatoes, nearly all the way through top to bottom, in six sections (scoop out tomato seeds)
4. Open tomatoes and stuff with chicken salad
5. Chill and serve on bed of lettuce

◾ COLE SLAW

Yield: 4 servings	Serving size: 1/2 cup
20 cal/serving .235g fat	% cal fat: 3%
carbo: 92%	protein: 5%

INGREDIENTS:

2 cups finely chopped cabbage
1 cup shredded carrot
1/4 cup red wine vinegar
1/2 teaspoon garlic powder
1 teaspoon celery seed
1/2 teaspoon ground pepper
2 tablespoons low-fat mayonnaise
artificial sweetener to taste

PROCEDURE:

1. Thoroughly mix all ingredients by hand
2. Chill before serving

◣ Crabmeat Salad

Yield: 4 servings	Serving size: 1 tomato or 3/4 cup (when used for sandwich)
160 cal/serving 1.91g fat carbo: 28%	% cal fat: 10% protein: 62%

INGREDIENTS:

16 ounces cooked, drained crabmeat
2 cups diced celery
juice of 2 lemons
4 tablespoons nonfat mayonnaise
white pepper to taste
4 whole medium tomatoes

PROCEDURE:

1. Gently mix crabmeat, celery, and lemon juice in a mixing bowl
2. Add mayonnaise and pepper
3. Slice tomato nearly all the way through top to bottom, in four sections, and scoop out seeds
4. Stuff tomatoes with crabmeat mixture
5. Chill before serving

◨ MACARONI SALAD

Yield: 4 servings	Serving size: 3/4 cup
118 cal/serving .583g fat	% cal fat: 4%
carbo: 83%	protein: 13%

INGREDIENTS:

4 ounces dry macaroni
1 stalk celery, diced
1 tablespoon grated carrot
1/4 cup diced onion
1 tablespoon diced pimento
8 halved cherry tomatoes
2 tablespoons low-fat mayonnaise

PROCEDURE:

1. Cook pasta al dente
2. Rinse and drain macaroni
3. Mix all ingredients in a bowl
4. Chill before serving

N PASTA PRIMAVERA

Yield: 4 servings	Serving size: 1 1/2 cups
180 cal/serving 2.72g fat	% cal fat: 14%
carbo: 70%	protein: 16%

INGREDIENTS:

6 ounces dry colored rotini pasta (3 cups cooked)
1/4 cup low-fat Italian dressing
1/2 cup green pepper sliced Julienne style
1/2 cup onion sliced Julienne style
1 cup raw broccoli cut into small pieces
2 tablespoons grated Parmesan cheese
1 cup diced yellow squash

PROCEDURE:

1. Cook pasta al dente
2. Toss all ingredients together
3. Chill and serve on lettuce leaf with a black olive for garnish

◧ PETER'S POTATO SALAD

Yield: 4 servings	*Serving size: 3/4 cup*
115 cal/serving .258g fat	*% cal fat: 2%*
carbo: 80%	*protein: 18%*

INGREDIENTS:

3 cups cooked, diced potatoes
4 hardboiled egg whites, diced small
1 stalk diced celery
1/4 cup diced onion
1/4 cup low-fat mayonnaise
1 teaspoon dry mustard
1 teaspoon celery seed
white pepper to taste
1 tablespoon red wine vinegar

PROCEDURE:

1. Combine all ingredients together and toss until well mixed
2. Chill and serve on a bed of lettuce
3. Sprinkle with paprika, if desired

◩ Tuna Salad

Yield: 4 servings	Serving size: 1/4 cup
50 cal/serving .239g fat	% cal fat: 4%
carbo: 21%	protein: 75%

INGREDIENTS:

1 (6 1/2-ounce) can water-packed tuna
1/4 cup diced celery
1/4 cup diced onion
3 tablespoons low-fat mayonnaise
1/4 teaspoon dried thyme

PROCEDURE:

1. Mix all ingredients together
2. Serve with tomato and cucumber slices

▧ TURKEY FRUIT SALAD

Yield: 4 servings	Serving size: 1 1/4 cup
155 cal/serving 2.42g fat	% cal fat: 14%
carbo: 40%	protein: 46%

INGREDIENTS:

8 ounces cooked, skinless turkey breast, diced
2 cups diced celery
1 cup diced pineapple (fresh or packed in natural juice)
1 cup sliced seedless red grapes
8 tablespoons low-fat mayonnaise
juice of 1 lemon

PROCEDURE:

1. Gently toss turkey, celery, pineapple and grapes in small bowl
2. Squeeze in lemon juice and add mayonnaise; toss gently
3. Chill and serve on a bed of lettuce

Potatoes and Rice

Potatoes

◪ Mashed Potatoes

Yield: 4 servings	*Serving size: 1 cup*
220 cal/serving .373g fat	*% cal fat: 2%*
carbo: 88%	*protein: 10%*

INGREDIENTS:

4 medium (8-ounce) baking potatoes
1/2 cup skim milk
2 teaspoons finely chopped onions
1 cup diced fresh mushrooms
2 teaspoons freshly chopped parsley
pepper to taste

PROCEDURE:

1. Peel potatoes and boil for 30 minutes
2. Mash potatoes and slowly blend in milk
3. Add onions, mushrooms, parsley, and mix well
4. Add pepper to taste and serve immediately

◪ Oven Fries

Yield: 4 servings	*Serving size: 4 strips*
124 cal/serving .113g fat	*% cal fat: 1%*
carbo: 91%	*protein: 8%*

INGREDIENTS:

2 medium (8-ounce) baking potatoes
vegetable spray

PROCEDURE:

1. Preheat oven to 400°
2. Cut potatoes lengthwise in eighths, then cut each slice in strips like French fries
3. Place on cookie sheet that has been sprayed with vegetable spray; bake in oven for 1/2 hour
4. Serve hot

◼ POTATO WITH BROCCOLI & CHEESE SAUCE

Yield: 4 servings	Serving size: 1/2 potato
246 cal/serving 5g fat	% cal fat: 19%
carbo: 64%	protein: 17%

INGREDIENTS:

4 (8-ounce) baking potatoes
4 cups chopped broccoli
1 cup skim milk
2 ounces Velveeta light
1 1/2 tablespoons cornstarch dissolved in 2 tablespoons water

PROCEDURE:

1. Bake the potatoes at 400° for 40 minutes
2. Steam the broccoli for 10 minutes
3. Bring milk and cheese to a simmer in a small sauce pan, whisking constantly so it doesn't scorch
4. Whisk in the cornstarch and bring back to a simmer while you continue whisking
5. Slice potatoes down the centers, open, and scoop out a little to help hold sauce

6. Add broccoli and pour 1/4 cup cheese sauce on each serving
7. Serve immediately

◼ SCALLOPED POTATOES

Yield: 4 servings	Serving size: 1/2 cup
180 cal/serving 1.21g fat	% cal fat: 6%
carbo: 78%	protein: 16%

INGREDIENTS:

2 medium (8-ounce) baking potatoes, peeled and sliced thin
1 1/4 cups skim milk
2 tablespoons grated Parmesan cheese
1 tablespoon flour
1 tablespoon Butter Buds
1 small diced fresh onion

PROCEDURE:

1. Preheat oven to 400°
2. Place sliced potatoes in baking dish sprayed with vegetable spray
3. Mix remaining ingredients together and pour over potatoes
4. Cover and bake for 45 minutes
5. Serve immediately

◼ STUFFED POTATO

Yield: 4 servings	Serving size: 1/2 potato
160 cal/serving 1.19g fat	% cal fat: 7%
carbo: 68%	protein: 25%

INGREDIENTS:

2 medium (8-ounce) baking potatoes
1 cup low-fat cottage cheese
2 teaspoons chopped chives

PROCEDURE:

1. Preheat oven to 400°
2. Bake potatoes for 40 minutes
3. Cut potatoes in half while hot and scoop out insides
4. Blend cottage cheese in blender to smooth consistency
5. Mix potatoes, cheese, and chives together
6. Bake at 350° for 20 minutes; serve hot

Rice

◼ BARLEY RICE PILAF

Yield: 8 servings	Serving size: 1/2 cup
100 cal/serving .8g fat	% cal fat: 7%
carbo: 82%	protein: 11%

INGREDIENTS:

1 cup diced onion
2 cloves minced garlic
vegetable spray
2 cups chicken stock (commercially prepared or use recipe on page 229)
1/2 cup brown rice
1/2 cup barley

PROCEDURE:

1. In medium sauce pan sprayed with vegetable spray, sauté onion and garlic for 10 minutes
2. Turn on high and add chicken stock
3. Bring stock to a boil and add the rice and barley
4. Lower to a slow boil on medium heat
5. Cover and cook for 45 minutes or until liquid is absorbed
6. Serve hot

◼ Curried Rice

Yield: 3 servings	Serving size: 1/2 cup
120 cal/serving 1.18g fat	% cal fat: 9%
carbo: 82%	protein: 9%

INGREDIENTS:

1/2 cup brown or wild rice
1/2 cup chicken stock (commercially prepared or use recipe on page 229)
1/2 cup water
1 teaspoon curry powder*

PROCEDURE:

1. Place all ingredients in a quart covered casserole dish
2. Bring to a boil, then reduce heat and simmer, covered, 30 minutes or until rice is fluffy

ALTERNATIVE: Bake in oven at 400° for 30 minutes

3. Serve hot

*If you don't like curry, use parsley or another favorite spice

▨ ORANGE RICE

Yield: 10 servings	Serving size: 1/2 cup
100 cal/serving .611g fat	% cal fat: 5%
carbo: 86%	protein: 9%

INGREDIENTS:

1/2 cup orange juice concentrate
3 1/2 cups water
1 tablespoon grated orange rind
1/2 cup diced onion
1/2 cup diced celery
1 teaspoon salt (optional)
2 cups rice blend (equal parts white and brown rice)

PROCEDURE:

1. Place all ingredients except rice in a medium sauce pan and bring to a boil
2. Add the rice and reduce heat
3. Cover and simmer for 40–50 minutes or until liquid is gone
4. Serve hot

▨ RICE BLEND

Yield: 4 servings	Serving size: 1/2 cup
138 cal/serving .03g fat	% cal fat: 9%
carbo: 79%	protein: 12%

INGREDIENTS:

1/2 cup brown rice
1/2 cup wild rice
2 cups chicken stock (commercially prepared or use recipe on p. 229)

PROCEDURE:

1. Bring chicken stock to a boil
2. Add rice and simmer, covered, on medium heat for 30–40 minutes
3. Serve hot

N SAFFRON RICE

Yield: 3 servings	Serving size: 1/2 cup
120 cal/serving .918g fat	% cal fat: 7%
carbo: 84%	protein: 9%

INGREDIENTS:

1/2 cup rice blend (half brown rice, half wild rice)
1 cup chicken stock
1/2 teaspoon saffron

PROCEDURE:

1. Bring chicken stock to boil in small sauce pan
2. Add saffron and rice, lower heat, and simmer, covered, for 20–25 minutes
3. Serve hot

Sauces and Stocks

◙ BARBECUE SAUCE

Yield: 1 cup	20 cal/tablespoon
.082g fat	% cal fat: 4%
carbo: 93%	protein: 3%

INGREDIENTS:

1 cup light tomato ketchup
juice of 1/2 lemon
1 tablespoon Worcestershire sauce
1 tablespoon white vinegar
1 clove garlic minced or pressed
1 bay leaf
1 teaspoon chili powder
1 tablespoon honey
1/2 teaspoon liquid smoke flavoring (optional)
2 tablespoons brown sugar

PROCEDURE:

1. Combine all ingredients in small sauce pan
2. Simmer for 1/2 hour, stirring frequently, until sauce
   thickens; use with meat, poultry, or fish

Ⓝ DILL SAUCE (FOR FISH)

Yield: 18 tablespoons	10 cal/tablespoon
.219g fat	% cal fat: 20%
carbo: 49%	protein: 31%

INGREDIENTS:

1 cup plain low-fat yogurt
2 tablespoons prepared horseradish
1 teaspoon dry mustard
1 tablespoon dried dill weed

PROCEDURE:

1. Mix all ingredients together by hand
2. Heat on low and serve hot

Ⓝ FLORENTINE SAUCE (FOR FISH)

Yield: 18 tablespoons	15 cal/tablespoon
.555g fat	% cal fat: 33%
carbo: 35%	protein: 14%

INGREDIENTS:

1 cup white sauce (recipe in this section)
1/4 cup dry white wine
dash hot sauce
1/4 teaspoon dried oregano
1/2 teaspoon dried dill weed
1/2 teaspoon white pepper
1/2 cup steamed spinach

PROCEDURE:

1. Combine first 6 ingredients and simmer for 2 minutes
2. Serve over fish and steamed spinach

▨ MINT SAUCE (FOR LAMB)

Yield: 1 cup	4 cal/tablespoon
0g fat	% cal fat: 0%
carbo: 100%	protein: 0%

INGREDIENTS:

1 cup white vinegar
1 tablespoon freshly chopped mint leaves
1 tablespoon cornstarch
low-calorie sweetener to taste

PROCEDURE:

1. Mix all ingredients together in a small sauce pan and simmer 15 minutes; serve hot

▨ ORANGE SAUCE (FOR POULTRY)

Yield: 3/4 cup	18 cal/tablespoon
.022g fat	% cal fat: 1%
carbo: 97%	protein: 2%

INGREDIENTS:

juice from 4 oranges or 1/2 cup orange juice
1 tablespoon grated orange peel
2 tablespoons honey
1 tablespoon cornstarch
2 tablespoons water

PROCEDURE:

1. Heat orange juice, orange peel, and honey in small sauce pan
2. Dissolve cornstarch in water
3. Add cornstarch to orange mixture and simmer for 5 minutes

◙ RAISIN SAUCE

Yield: 1 cup	27 cal/tablespoon
.04g fat	% cal fat: 2%
carbo: 96%	protein: 2%

INGREDIENTS:

1 cup cider
1/2 cup raisins
1 tablespoon sherry
1 teaspoon grated lemon rind
1/2 teaspoon prepared mustard
1 teaspoon sugar
2 tablespoons cornstarch
1/4 cup cold water

PROCEDURE:

1. Mix all ingredients, except cornstarch, in a small sauce pan and bring to a simmer
2. Dissolve cornstarch in water
3. Blend cornstarch into the sauce and simmer for 4–5 minutes or until thickened
4. Serve hot

◪ TOMATO SAUCE

Yield: 5 cups	110 cal/cup
1.31g fat	% cal fat: 11%
carbo: 75%	protein: 14%

INGREDIENTS:

10 medium tomatoes
1 cup diced onion
8 cloves minced garlic
1/4 cup beef stock (commercially prepared or recipe on page 228)
3 teaspoons dried oregano
1 tablespoon dried basil
1 bay leaf
1 teaspoon dried thyme
black pepper to taste
1/2 cup low-sodium tomato paste
1/4 cup Burgundy wine
artificial sweetener to taste

PROCEDURE:

1. Place tomatoes in a pot, cover with water, and heat until skins loosen
2. Peel tomatoes and puree in blender; place tomatoes in heavy sauce pot
3. Simmer onions, garlic, beef stock in nonstick skillet
4. Add onion mixture and spices to tomatoes, cover, and simmer on medium heat for 1/2 hour
5. Add tomato paste and wine and simmer for 1/2 hour; serve hot

◼ BEEF STOCK

Yield: 2 quarts	50 cal/cup
1g fat	% cal fat: 18%
carbo: 42%	protein: 40%

INGREDIENTS:

1 cup + 2 quarts water
3 carrots cut into quarters
3 celery stalks cut into quarters
1 quartered medium onion
2 pounds beef bones

PROCEDURE:

1. Preheat oven to 450°
2. Pour 1 cup water into roasting pan; add vegetables and bones
3. Bake until bones brown, approximately 1 to 2 hours, mixing occasionally
4. Remove from oven and pour all ingredients into a stockpot or sauce pan
5. Add 2 quarts water into roasting pan and bring to boil on top of stove, scraping everything off the sides and bottom
6. Pour everything into stockpot and simmer uncovered for 2 hours
7. Strain through colander or cheesecloth
8. Refrigerate
9. After stock cools, remove fat before using

NOTE: May be frozen

▧ CHICKEN STOCK

Yield: 2 quarts	30 cal/cup
.5g fat	% cal fat: 15%
carbo: 35%	protein: 50%

INGREDIENTS:

3 pounds leftover chicken parts (neck, wings, bones, etc.)
2 quartered medium onions
4 celery stalks cut in quarters
4 carrots cut in quarters
1 bay leaf
2 quarts water
2 egg shells

PROCEDURE:

1. Place all ingredients in stockpot and simmer, covered, for 2 hours
2. Strain through colander or cheesecloth
3. Refrigerate
4. After stock cools, remove fat before using

NOTE: May be frozen

Desserts, Minimeals
and Breakfasts

◪ BAKED APPLE

Yield: 4 servings	Serving size: 1 apple
100 cal/serving 1.42g fat	% cal fat: 13%
carbo: 85%	protein: 2%

INGREDIENTS:

4 fresh apples (approximately 7 ounces each)
4 teaspoons ground cinnamon
4 teaspoons ground nutmeg

PROCEDURE:

1. Preheat oven to 350°
2. Core apples
3. Place cinnamon and nutmeg in the core hollows
4. Bake uncovered for 30 minutes
5. Serve warm

(OPTION: Add yogurt or raisins after baking)

N FRUIT AMBROSIA

Yield: 4 servings	Serving size: 2/3 cup
100 cal/serving .426g fat	% cal fat: 4%
carbo: 91%	protein: 5%

INGREDIENTS:
juice of 1 lemon
1/2 finely chopped apple
1/2 finely chopped orange
1/2 finely chopped grapefruit
8 seedless grapes
1/4 finely chopped honeydew
1/4 finely chopped cantaloupe
grated coconut

PROCEDURE:
1. Combine ingredients in mixing bowl and chill
2. Lightly sprinkle each serving with grated coconut
   before chilling

N FRUIT PARFAIT

Yield: 4 servings	Serving size: 1 parfait
100 cal/serving .992g fat	% cal fat: 9%
carbo: 72%	protein: 19%

INGREDIENTS:
2 packages low-calorie (no sugar) strawberry gelatin
2 whole ripe bananas, quartered
2 cups strawberries, quartered
1/2 cup low-fat plain yogurt

PROCEDURE:

1. Prepare gelatin according to directions on package
2. Layer ingredients in each parfait glass as follows:
   1/4 cup gelatin
   1/4 banana
   1/4 cup strawberries
   1 tablespoon yogurt
   1/4 cup gelatin
   1/4 banana
   1/4 cup strawberries
   1 tablespoon yogurt
3. To serve, chill and garnish with fresh strawberry or mint leaf

◧ High Fiber Cookies

Yield: 24 2 1/2" cookies	55 cal/cookie
1.08g fat	% cal fat: 18%
carbo: 65%	protein: 17%

INGREDIENTS:
4 egg whites
1 tablespoon low-fat corn-oil margarine
1/3 cup granulated sugar
3/4 cup skim milk
2 teaspoons vanilla extract
1/2 teaspoon salt
1 cup oat bran
1 cup whole wheat flour
1 cup oatmeal
2 teaspoons ground cinnamon
1/2 teaspoon baking soda
1/2 teaspoon baking powder

PROCEDURE:

1. Preheat oven to 350°
2. Cream together eggs, margarine, and sugar
3. Add milk, vanilla, salt, and beat until smooth
4. Mix remaining dry ingredients together, then blend with liquid ingredients
5. Drop by teaspoon on baking sheet and bake for 8–10 minutes

NOTE: May add 1/2 cup raisins for different texture

▧ OATMEAL COOKIES

Yield: 18 cookies	96 cal/cookie
3.67g fat	% cal fat: 34%
carbo: 56%	protein: 10%

INGREDIENTS:

1/3 cup brown sugar
1/2 cup all-purpose flour
1/2 cup oat bran
1 1/2 cups "quick" rolled oats
1/2 teaspoon baking soda
1/2 teaspoon salt
1/2 teaspoon baking powder
1/4 cup sugar
1/4 cup canola oil
4 egg whites
1 teaspoon vanilla extract

PROCEDURE:

1. Preheat oven to 400°

2. Mix all dry (first eight) ingredients in one bowl; mix all liquids (next three) in another
3. Combine dry and liquid ingredients; mix with a wooden spoon
4. Using 2 tablespoons of mixture per cookie, place on nonstick baking sheet
5. Bake for 8–10 minutes
6. Add 1/2 cup raisins for different texture

◻ FRENCH TOAST

Yield: 4 slices	Serving size: 1 slice
127 cal/slice 1.13g fat	% cal fat: 8%
carbo: 58%	protein: 34%

INGREDIENTS:

1 cup Egg Beaters®
1/4 cup skim or 1/2% milk
2 teaspoons cinnamon
1 teaspoon vanilla extract
vegetable spray
4 slices low calorie wheat or regular bread

PROCEDURE:

1. Combine Egg Beaters®, milk, cinnamon, and vanilla in a bowl
2. Beat with a whisk
3. Heat Teflon pan or griddle
4. Spray pan with vegetable spray
5. Coat bread with egg mixture and fry on each side until browned
6. Serve with low calorie syrup

Chapter 19
◪ ◪ ◪
A FINAL WORD

Now that you know about the New Hilton Head Metabolism Diet, get started right away. A new body and a new metabolism await you. Don't put it off. This diet has worked for thousands and thousands of others and it can work for you too.

The closer you stick to my recommendations, the better you will do. Make certain you:

1. Begin with the Weekday Low-Calorie and Weekend Booster Stages
2. Use Dietary Stairstepping to switch to the Maintenance Stage after four to six weeks of dieting
3. Eat three meals and two minimeals a day
4. Schedule two Thermal Walks every day
5. Schedule the Muscle Firmers three times a week
6. Practice Willpower Training to keep you from succumbing to out-of-control eating

Don't leave out any of these basic elements. Try not to modify the basic plan or it may not work as well for you.

Before you know it, you'll look and feel totally different. You'll have a slimmer figure, a firmer body, and a more efficient metabolism. And best of all, you'll be in control of your eating and successfully managing your weight for years to come.

◪ ◪ ◪
ABOUT THE AUTHOR

Peter M. Miller, Ph.D., founded the Hilton Head Health Institute in 1976 and is its executive director.

Dr. Miller received a bachelor of arts degree from the University of Maryland and a doctorate in clinical psychology from the University of South Carolina. He holds a faculty appointment in the Department of Health Education at the University of South Carolina and is the author of ten books and more than sixty research articles. He is also the editor in chief of the scientific journal, *Addictive Behaviors*, which publishes studies on obesity, smoking, alcoholism, and drug abuse.

Under his leadership the Institute has developed an international reputation in the treatment of weight problems and has been ranked one of the top five health resorts in the world. Offering a highly effective, long-term plan to overcome the metabolic and psychological barriers to successful weight control, the Institute's various programs have some of the highest success rates of any facility of its type.

The Hilton Head Health Institute offers one- to four-week programs, refresher courses, and weekend escapes on weight control, smoking cessation and stress management. Its campus on semitropical Hilton Head Island, South Carolina, offers a secluded retreat with a daily program schedule that balances time for learning and reflection with exercise and recreation.

For more information about the Hilton Head Health Institute and its programs, write the author at:

Dr. Peter M. Miller
The Hilton Head Health Institute
P.O. Box 7138
Hilton Head Island, SC 29938-7138

Or call toll-free:

From the USA: 1-800-292-2440
From Canada: 1-800-348-2039

INDEX

N N N

RECIPE INDEX